Defining Death

DEFINING
DEATH

The Case for Choice

ROBERT M. VEATCH
and
LAINIE F. ROSS

Georgetown University Press / Washington, DC

Library of Congress Cataloging-in-Publication Data
Names: Veatch, Robert M., author. | Ross, Lainie Friedman, author.
Title: Defining death : the case for choice / by Robert M. Veatch, Lainie Friedman Ross.
Description: Washington, DC : Georgetown University Press, 2016. | Includes bibliographical references and index.
Identifiers: LCCN 2016001904 (print) | LCCN 2016006088 (ebook) | ISBN 9781626163546 (hc : alk. paper) | ISBN 9781626163553 (pb : alk. paper) | ISBN 9781626163560 (eb)
Subjects: LCSH: Death. | Brain death.
Classification: LCC RA1063 .V43 2016 (print) | LCC RA1063 (ebook) | DDC 616.07/8—dc23
LC record available at http://lccn.loc.gov/2016001904

∞ This book is printed on acid-free paper meeting the requirements of the American National Standard for Permanence in Paper for Printed Library Materials.

17 16   9 8 7 6 5 4 3 2 First printing

Printed in the United States of America

Cover design by Anne C. Kerns, Anne Likes Red, Inc.

For

Ann B. Veatch

and

John L. Ross

*with gratitude and affection
for sharing the journey*

CONTENTS

1

Defining Death: An Introduction

There was a day when everyone could tell the difference between the living and the dead. Over the past fifty years, that has changed. Of course, occasional mistakes in pronouncing death have always occurred—when a physician could not feel a pulse and pronounced a patient dead only to have the heart start again. Occasionally, the patient recovered enough to survive and leave the hospital. The physician might have said something like, "I thought the patient had died, but I was mistaken." Sometimes the one making the statement might say something a bit different. He or she might say, "The patient died and came back to life." Thoughtful commentators have always understood that this is not correct. There is one death per person, at least in this world. The more accurate observation would be something like, "The patient suffered a cardiac arrest that we thought was irreversible, but obviously it was not. He would have died had not the heart started beating again." The difference is critical because many important clinical, social, legal, and personal issues are at stake when we pronounce someone dead. The spouse becomes a widow; the person's assets are disposed of; health insurance coverage stops (health insurance does not cover dead people). On the other hand, life insurance pays off; the will is executed; if the deceased is president of a country, he or she ceases to be president, and a successor assumes the office. In medicine important implications follow as well. Not only does medical treatment to preserve life cease, but organs can be procured.

The Emergence of the Controversy

Until about the middle of the twentieth century, this all seemed straightforward. The doctor (or even a layperson) could feel the pulse, listen for the heartbeat, or in the classic movie scene, place a mirror to the nostrils to see if the person was breathing and, on this basis, decide whether someone was dead or alive. We knew that in some special cases, determining that circulation had stopped (and especially determining that it had stopped permanently) was a bit difficult for the layperson, so we generally relied on physicians or other health professionals in cases that were not obvious. But no one questioned exactly what it meant to be dead or alive.

Then about that time we began to develop new technologies and medical interventions that could stretch out the dying process and permit us to ask more precisely what it was about the bodily changes occurring that should be treated as the event we call death. Mechanical ventilators, heart-lung machines, dialysis machines, the techniques of cardiopulmonary resuscitation, extracorporeal membrane oxygenation, artificial hearts, left ventricular assist devices (LVADs), and other technologies made it possible to ask exactly what event should be called "death."

In 1959 a French publication introduced the term *le coma dépassé* (roughly, overwhelming or deep coma), and suggestions were made that people in such a condition were, in effect, dead.[1] Spurred on by advances in organ transplantation, an American committee based at Harvard Medical School published a report in 1968 that also connected irreversible brain function loss to death. Titled "A Definition of Irreversible Coma," the report provided criteria for measuring what it called "irreversible coma" and claimed that this state was what should be considered death.[2] We shall see that, while the report provided diagnostic criteria for this condition, it really did not argue why these criteria should replace the traditional circulatory and respiratory criteria. Very soon thereafter, however, states, beginning with Kansas in 1970,[3] began changing their laws so that death could be pronounced on the basis of irreversible loss of brain function in addition to the traditional criteria focusing on circulation.

Within a very short period, scholars working with this literature began to realize that being in a coma, even a "permanent or irreversible" coma,[4] was not exactly the same as losing all functions of the brain. By 1971 neurologists knew that one could be in what appeared to be an irreversible coma without meeting the Harvard criteria (as they began to be called).[5] Eventually, it was evident that certain functions of the brain could remain when the Harvard criteria were met.[6]

Three Groups of Definitions

The result was an increasingly complicated set of views about what it took to be called "dead." One group held that a human is dead when there is irreversible loss of functions of the entire brain (including the brain stem). Another smaller group consisted of a persistent hard core of defenders of circulatory-based concepts of death. Members of this group insisted that we should revert to more traditional criteria for pronouncing death. A third group also began to emerge. Its members held that only certain brain functions were critical as an indicator of life. They were a diverse group with members that thought somewhat different functions were critical. Thus, for example, some held that as long as someone was in an irreversible coma, that person should be classified as dead even if some "trivial" functions, such as brain-stem reflexes, remained. Thus, three clusters of concepts of death competed in the public discourse: one based on irreversible loss of all brain functions that has been referred to as "whole-brain function"; one based on irreversible loss of circulatory function; and one based on loss of what came ambiguously to be called "higher-brain function," usually equated with consciousness.

Moreover, within each of these three clusters of definitions of death were countless variations. For those supporting the whole-brain concept of death, some insisted that literally every function of the brain must be lost for death to occur whereas others excluded some minor, or "trivial," functions like an auditory nerve potential or certain hormone secretions. For those supporting the cardiocirculatory concept, some equated death with the permanent stoppage of the heart, but since circulation can now be maintained with heart-lung machines, LVADs, or artificial hearts, others equated it with permanent loss of circulation. For those supporting the higher-brain view, some would insist on loss of all cerebral activity; others only on loss of consciousness.

In short, there are many, many different concepts of death that have thoughtful people as advocates. It is now apparent that even if we limit our attention to a single country, like the United States, no concept of death is supported by the majority of the population. Moreover, in different countries different concepts of death have different levels of support.

The Emergence of a Uniform Brain-Oriented Definition

The US President's Commission for the Study of Ethical Problems in Medicine and Biomedical and Behavioral Research, which was established in 1978, recognized the need for a uniform definition of death. The commission's report, *Defining Death*, was published in 1981. The commission had three aims: "1) to provide a conceptual basis for the new medical practice of death determination using neurological tests; 2) to explain the relationship between determining death on neurological and circulatory-respiratory grounds; and 3) to enhance the uniformity among jurisdictions by proposing and justifying a model statute, the Uniform Determination of Death Act (UDDA)."[7] The report did an excellent job in fulfilling these three aims, and the Uniform Law Commissioners, the American Bar Association (ABA), and the American Medical Association (AMA) approved the model statute as a substitute for their previous proposals. The statute was also endorsed by the American Academy of Neurology (AAN) and the American Electroencephalographic Society.[8]

The model statute stated,

§ 1. [*Determination of Death.*] An individual who has sustained either (1) irreversible cessation of circulatory and respiratory functions, or (2) irreversible cessation of all functions of the entire brain, including the brain stem, is dead. A determination of death must be made in accordance with accepted medical standards.

§ 2. [*Uniformity of Construction and Application.*] This act shall be applied and construed to effectuate its general purpose to make uniform the law with respect to the subject of this Act among states enacting it.

Irreversible versus Permanent Loss of Function

Probably the biggest controversy left in the wake of the report was that it used the terms "permanent loss of function" and "irreversible loss of function" interchangeably, although the model statute only used the word "irreversible." There is a possible difference between "permanent" loss of function and "irreversible" loss. Loss that is "permanent" will never be restored, even though medically it could be if appropriate interventions took place. On the other hand, loss that is "irreversible" could not be restored, even if someone tried as aggressively as possible to restore it.

James Bernat, a Dartmouth physician and a strong proponent of the UDDA, argues that "permanent and irreversible cessation of functions are distinct phenomena but are related causally. All functions that are irreversibly lost are also permanently lost (but not vice versa)."[9] However, he argues that permanent cessation of function is a valid surrogate for irreversible cessation when resuscitation will not be performed, thereby empowering physicians to make a more timely determination of death.[10] The need for timeliness is intertwined with organ transplantation. That is, one can distinguish between physiological irreversibility (cannot be restored) and legal or moral irreversibility (one will not attempt restoration because the person has refused resuscitation such that cessation is permanent).[11]

Defining Death and Transplanting Organs

The historical connection between this discussion of the definition of death and organ transplantation seems inescapable. Several months before the Harvard Ad Hoc Committee report was published, the Uniform Anatomical Gift Act (UAGA), which allowed for organ donation, had been passed.[12] The Harvard Committee pointed out the advantage for procurement of organs if some humans could be classified as deceased while, supported by a ventilator, circulation and cardiac function remained to perfuse the organs. Assuming we cannot take life-prolonging organs until someone is dead (what is usually called the "dead donor rule"), it is not only crucial to know exactly when someone dies; it is also advantageous if something other than circulatory loss signals death. The article that followed the Harvard Committee's report in *JAMA* (the *Journal of the American Medical Association*) was by the American Medical Association Judicial Council and was titled "Ethical Guidelines for Organ Transplantation."[13]

In spite of the obvious connection between the definition of death and organ transplantation, others have insisted that we should not be able to tailor-make a definition of death for various purposes such as organ procurement. A single definition should apply to all regardless of the usefulness of a particular definition for special cases. If death in humans is the irreversible loss of what is essential to being human, it seems reasonable that some set of functions controlled by the brain is as essential—perhaps more essential—than a mere pump and set of tubes in which blood flows. But if this is true, it should be true regardless of whether we contemplate organ procurement following death. It is intrinsically important that we know whether a person with a beating heart and a dead brain is dead or alive, even if that person could not possibly be a donor of organs. Moreover, if it turns out to be implausible to insist that every last function of a brain be lost irreversibly in order to pronounce death, it is also important to know which brain functions can be ignored. Thus, the definition of death is an important question independent of organ transplantation as well as for determining which organ procurements conform to the dead donor rule.

The Structure of the Book

This significant, if not exclusive, connection between defining death and organ transplantation led us to devote the first third of our book *Transplantation Ethics*, 2nd edition, to the defining of death. At the same time, we recognize that many people are interested in the definition-of-death question even if they are not directly interested in transplantation. Thus, we have decided to publish as a freestanding short book a volume based on the first part of our work exploring the ethics of transplantation. We hope it will be useful to neurologists and other health professionals as well as to lawyers and other public policy proponents. It should serve a purpose for philosophers, theologians, and those studying the ethics of health care when they contemplate the decision to withhold or withdraw life-sustaining treatment. In particular, it should speak to when it is no longer possible to decide to forgo life-sustaining treatment because the patient is no longer with us. Most people today do not believe that life support must always be provided just because the patient is alive, but most continue to believe that there is normally no reason to provide medical treatment for the dead. (There may be temporary exceptions if a body is to be preserved for organ procurement or research or, in rare instances, to function as an environment for a previable fetus.) Health insurance, for example, should not normally pay for continuing treatments on the dead body. More critically, families need to know when it is time to begin the grieving process that accompanies the pronouncement of death.

The structure of the remaining six chapters of the book is as follows. In chapter 2 we explore the dead donor rule—a major catalyst for the debate surrounding when a person is classified as dead—and some basic conceptual issues. We then devote a chapter to each of the three main clusters of concepts of death (the whole-brain concept, the circulatory concept, and the higher-brain concept). We shall develop the claim that there are many variant positions within each of the three main concepts. We conclude that there are no definitive, scientific arguments to support any one of these three main concepts. When one takes into account the countless variations within the three main concepts, it seems increasingly clear that no one definition of death can command anything approaching a simple majority support, let alone a consensus.

We argue that choosing a definition of death for public policy and other social purposes is, in fact, a philosophical, religious, or social choice. We should pick the definition that produces the most consistent and reasonable implications for how we should treat people. We are, in effect, trying to identify the moment at which society should decide that someone is no longer with us and that we should treat that person the way we treat the dead. Our claim is that the choice of a definition of death is not a scientific one but a social one. We claim that the choice should be handled the way society handles other religious, philosophical, or social choices. We should give people some space to make personal, conscientious choices among plausible definitions. Since not everyone will make an explicit choice among the major concepts of death, society needs a default in order to know how to proceed, but individuals should also have a range of discretion in picking an alternative definition based on their personal beliefs and values.

We thus, in the sixth chapter, make a case for a public policy that establishes one definition as a default. That seems necessary to avoid the public policy chaos of having no way to deal with a patient who has no known preference for a particular definition. However, we propose that, since choosing among these definitions of death necessarily relies on basic religious and philosophical beliefs about what is essential to human existence and that such matters are often left to conscience, individuals who object to the default definition should be permitted to pick an alternative. Since some extreme choices might lead to public health problems or to moral concerns about treating respiring, thinking, conscious humans as dead, we propose that there must be some reasonable limits to conscientious choice of a definition, but any choice from among the three main concepts of death seems tolerable.

To those who complain that permitting such choice could create serious social disutilities, we examine some alternative ways of dealing with those disutilities. For example, if someone opts for a traditional circulatory concept of death and ends up stable in a coma, potentially of many years' duration, and if this happened often enough that it imposed severe economic impact on others in the same health insurance pool, we could require that those who opt for the circulatory definition also buy an insurance rider at market rates to cover those costs. It seems likely that the number of people opting for that definition and then ending up in a coma that is medically stable for a long duration is so small that the costs would not be a serious issue. Our point is that there are alternatives for dealing with most, if not all, the social and economic issues that could arise with a policy of permitting people to conscientiously dissent from the default definition of death.

Similarly, if someone opts for a higher-brain definition of death, that person could be declared dead sooner than those preferring either of the other definitions. That could impose a problem for life insurance companies. These same people (or their surrogates), however, already have the right to refuse life-supporting medical treatment and increasingly they have the option of refusing nutrition and hydration or even choosing physician-assisted suicide. Once they reach a condition in which critical cerebral function is permanently lost, they might be dead soon anyway, having opted to forgo life support or making other critical choices (or having their surrogates make these choices for them). Either way, the public impact of opting for an alternative definition of death is likely to be minimal, or so we argue in chapter 6.

Finally, in the last chapter we propose a new definition-of-death law, one that relies on the now widely accepted language of the brain-based death laws but that adds a morally critical conscience clause permitting people to opt for an alternative definition of death for their own death pronouncement.

What appears is essentially part 1 of *Transplantation Ethics*, 2nd edition. We had at first anticipated only minor updating and editing. We have discovered, however, that the debate over the definition of death is a very rapidly moving field. Since the publication of *Transplantation Ethics*, 2nd edition, a great deal has happened. Two important legal cases have raised serious questions about the viability of a neurological definition of death. One of these, the case of Jahi McMath, was just emerging when we published the transplantation volume. We had no idea that Jahi's bodily functions would be maintained for over two years even though three sets of competent neurologists and at least one court and one medical examiner had ruled she was dead. Now, not only have her bodily functions been maintained but her family has claimed that her brain is still functioning, leading them to demand that the court for the first time ever reverse the death declaration. Meanwhile, in another case, that of a young woman named Aden Hailu, the Nevada Supreme Court intervened to prevent doctors from pronouncing Hailu dead even though she met the most widely accepted brain-based criteria for death. We introduce both of these cases in chapter 3 and tease out some potentially radical—indeed shocking—implications. Even if these two cases are resolved in the near future, we can now anticipate more controversies raising the issues they have introduced.

We have also been able to add a surprising number of new references that have become available since the appearance of *Transplantation Ethics*, 2nd edition. We have further clarified a number of the arguments and issues. We hope these changes, which sometimes turn out to be more than modest, contribute to the provocatively rich discussion of what it means to be dead.

In sum we hope that providing a small volume on the current state of the definition-of-death debate serves a useful purpose for those who are interested in the controversies surrounding the definition, determination, and declaration of death even if they are not interested in pursuing the ethics of procuring or allocating organs for transplant.

Notes

1. Mollaret P, Goulon M, "Le coma dépassé," *Revue Neurologique* 1959;103:3–15.

2. Harvard Medical School Ad Hoc Committee, "A definition of irreversible coma. Report of the Ad Hoc Committee of the Harvard Medical School to Examine the Definition of Brain Death," *JAMA* 1968;205(6):337–340.

3. Kansas Statutes Annotated, § 77–202 (sup. 1971).

4. Death is delineated in the Uniform Determination of Death Act (UDDA), defined later in the chapter, as irreversible loss of function, although for most declarations of death, physicians evaluate only for permanent loss of function. (See Bernat JL, Capron AM, Bleck TP, et al., "The circulatory-respiratory determination of death in organ donation," *Critical Care Medicine* 2010;38[3]:963–970.) We discuss the difference between permanent and irreversible later in the chapter.

5. Brierley JB, Adam JAH, Graham DI, Simpson JA, "Neocortical death after cardiac arrest," *Lancet* 1971;2(7224):560–565.

6. Halevy A, Brody B, "Brain death: reconciling definitions, criteria, and tests," *Annals of Internal Medicine* 1993;119(6):519–525.

7. Bernat et al., "Circulatory-respiratory determination," 963–964.

8. President's Commission for the Study of Ethical Problems in Medicine and Biomedical and Behavioral Research, *Defining Death: Medical, Legal and Ethical Issues in the Determination of Death* (Washington, DC: US Government Printing Office, July 1981), 73.

9. Bernat JL, "How the distinction between 'irreversible' and 'permanent' illuminates circulatory-respiratory death determination," *Journal of Medicine and Philosophy* 2010;35(3):246.

10. Ibid.

11. See, for example, Tomlinson T, "The irreversibility of death: reply to Cole," *Kennedy Institute of Ethics Journal* 1993;3(2):157–165;

Marquis D, "Are DCD donors dead?" *Hastings Center Report* 2010; 40(3):24–31.

12. Uniform Anatomical Gift Act (UAGA) 1968.

13. American Medical Association Judicial Council, "Ethical guidelines for organ transplantation," *JAMA* 1968;205(6):341–342.

2

The Dead Donor Rule
and the Concept of Death

On May 25, 1968, at the beginning of the era of transplantation, Bruce Tucker was brought to the operating room of the hospital of the Medical College of Virginia in Richmond. Tucker, a fifty-six-year-old black laborer, had suffered a massive brain injury the day before in a fall. He had sustained a lateral basilar skull fracture on the right side, a subdural hematoma on the left side, and brain-stem contusion. The case revealed the complexities of deciding when and which criteria to use to declare a patient dead and legitimately procure organs for transplantation. It eventually ended up in the Virginia courts.

According to a timetable summarized by Judge A. Christian Compton, who eventually heard the case when it came to court, Tucker was admitted to the hospital at 6:05 p.m. An emergency right temporoparietal craniotomy was performed, and a right parietal burr hole was drilled.[1] Tucker was placed on a respirator, which kept him "mechanically alive." The treating physician noted that his "prognosis for recovery is nil and death imminent." By 1:00 p.m. the next day, the neurologist had called to obtain an electroencephalogram (EEG), and the results showed "flat lines with occasional artifact. He found no clinical evidence of viability and no evidence of cortical activity."

At 2:45 p.m. Tucker was taken to the operating room. According to the court record, "he maintained vital signs of life, that is, he maintained, for the most part, normal body temperature, normal pulse, normal blood pressure and normal rate of respiration." At 3:30 p.m. the respirator was cut off, and the patient was pronounced dead. His heart and kidneys were removed for transplanting.

The Tucker case was the first widely publicized controversy about the question of when a person is dead. Many interpret the case as establishing a brain-oriented definition of death for the state of Virginia, but it could equally be viewed as the first case in which a ventilator was disconnected for the purpose of causing the death of the patient, by traditional heart criteria, in order to procure organs for transplantation.

Tucker's brother, William Tucker, apparently saw it in this second way. He sued for $100,000 in damages, charging that the transplant team was engaged in a "systematic and nefarious scheme to use Bruce Tucker's heart and hastened his death by shutting off the mechanical means of support." Moreover, the organs were apparently procured with only minimal effort to locate the next of kin to obtain permission either to stop the respirator or to procure the organs. There were insinuations that the transplant team was quicker to act because the patient was black (and it does not help that the recipient was white). It might be worth noting that William Tucker's attorney was a young black Virginia state senator, L. Douglas Wilder, who later became the state's governor and a nationally known Democratic politician. The result of the legal case was ambiguous. The doctors were exonerated, but it is unclear whether the court held that the doctors had the authority to turn off the ventilator on a still-living patient in these circumstances or whether it held that Tucker was already dead according to brain criteria. Virginia's definition of death did not change as a result of the case.

In those early years of the definition-of-death debate and the organ transplant controversy, this case was one of the most complicated and significant. Whether it should in fact be treated as a "brain death" case is unclear, but certainly that is the way the principals in the case and the press handled it. *Internal Medicine News* headed its report "'Brain Death' Held Proof of Demise in Va. Jury Decision."[2]

The *New York Times*'s headline said, "Virginia Jury Rules That Death Occurs When Brain Dies."[3]

The surgeons who removed Bruce Tucker's heart evidently also interpreted the court ruling as deciding when a patient is dead. David Hume, the assisting surgeon in the case, is quoted as saying that the court's decision in favor of the physicians "brings the law up to date with what medicine has known all along—that the only death is brain death."

Most people assumed that, asked to decide whether the physicians were guilty of causing the death of the heart donor, the jury in the Tucker case was in effect being asked to make a public policy judgment about whether the irreversible loss of brain function should be equated for moral, legal, and public policy purposes with the death of an individual. Because almost all organs for transplant except for those from living kidney donors come from the bodies of the newly deceased and getting those organs in a viable condition is usually assumed to require getting them as soon after death as possible, it is critical to be clear on exactly what it means for a human to be dead.

It is possible that the court found the physicians' behavior acceptable because it believed that Tucker's brain had irreversibly stopped functioning and that this "death" of the brain should, contrary to what was then Virginia law, be the basis for pronouncing the person dead. It is also possible, however, that the members of the jury approved of the physicians' behavior because they believed that it was acceptable to stop the ventilator and let him die (on the basis of the stopping of heart function). Tucker's case would then be what we now would call a donation after circulatory death.

The case leaves many questions unanswered in addition to the issues related to the lack of consent for procuring organs. Why, for example, should a single flat-line EEG reading be taken as evidence of the irreversible loss of brain function? The events of the Tucker case occurred days after the publication of the Harvard Ad Hoc Committee's famous report that proposed the first peer-reviewed criteria for measuring the death of the brain.[4] A single flat EEG reading would not be sufficient by Harvard committee standards or any set of criteria published since then. Also, if Tucker was believed to be dead by brain function loss sometime before 3:30 p.m., why was the respirator turned off at that time? Unless one feels a need to pronounce death by heart function loss, it makes no sense to turn off the respirator on a man who is a candidate for organ procurement. If death is based on brain function loss, he was already dead before the respirator was stopped.

This case shows how confusing the early days were for pronouncing the deaths of severely brain-injured patients who were potential sources of organs for transplant. It reveals that we needed to do a great deal of work to understand precisely what it means to be dead in a context where someone envisions medical use of a body and where that use is acceptable only once the individual is considered deceased.

The task of defining death is not a trivial exercise in coining the meaning of a term. Rather, it is an attempt to reach an understanding of the philosophical nature of the human being and what it is that is essentially significant to humans that is lost at the time of death. When we say that an individual has died, there are appropriate behavioral changes: We go into mourning, perhaps cease certain kinds of medical treatment, initiate a funeral ritual, read a will, or if the individual happens to be president of an organization, elevate the vice president to the presidency. According to many, including those who focus on the definition of death as crucial for the transplant debate, it is appropriate to remove vital, unpaired organs after, but not before, death. This is what is usually called the "dead donor rule." So there is a great deal at stake at the policy level in the definition of death. We can start by examining this rule.

The Dead Donor Rule

The dead donor rule holds that a human being must be dead before life-prolonging organs (e.g., the heart, liver, or lungs) can be procured for transplantation or other purposes. This would exclude procuring a single kidney or a lobe of the liver, either of which would not be expected to end the life of the one from whom the part was taken. The dead donor rule has been discussed in the organ procurement literature for at least the past twenty-five years.[5]

The Standard View

At least until recently, almost everyone accepted this rule. People might have disagreed about exactly what it means to be dead, but there has been a widespread consensus that life-prolonging organs can be procured only once death has occurred. Otherwise, the one procuring these organs would cause the death of the one who is the source of the organs. The organ provider would be killed by means of organ procurement. And the intentional killing of an innocent human, even for the good cause of saving the lives of others, has been almost universally viewed as both unethical and illegal. Some with more radical views would even extend the prohibition on killing to cases of war and self-defense, but almost everyone has assumed that innocent people should not be killed intentionally. This includes the killing of those near an inevitable death, even if they give their permission. Just as the intentional killing of another for mercy has almost universally been unacceptable in medicine, so too killing for purposes of procuring organs has been condemned.

The Challenge

Recently, a number of critics have challenged the dead donor rule. Some are concerned that organs will deteriorate unnecessarily if the person who is to be the source of the organs has a respirator stopped or otherwise goes through a process whereby the procurement team waits for the death to occur before intervening. Most of the critics argue a more principled case. They claim that it ought not to be considered immoral to kill patients under certain circumstances, particularly when they are terminally ill and give their permission to have their lives terminated.

This is essentially the position of those who, outside the context of organ procurement, are now defending active, intentional killing—often called euthanasia or physician-assisted suicide. It stands to reason that those who favor euthanasia would be open to killing by means of organ removal in cases where they found other means of euthanasia acceptable. A group of scholars and activists has, during the past two decades or more, been pressing their case for the morality, and sometimes even the legalization, of such killings.[6] For now, however, professional groups, academics, and religious bodies in the United States have for the most part remained opposed to these efforts.[7]

Since the late twentieth century, however, a small group of serious scholars has endorsed the procurement of organs without waiting for death to be pronounced, although they have not necessarily taken a position on the broader question of intentional killings for mercy.[8] Robert Truog, as a coauthor with Franklin Miller and Dan Brock, has argued in favor of procurement before death pronouncement in cases where the patient has consented to withdrawal of life support and has agreed to donate organs.[9] Truog and his colleagues first claim, correctly, that even with the withdrawal of life support, the physician who withdraws the life-supporting intervention plays a role in the causal chain leading to the patient's death.

They then claim that if a valid consent is obtained, there is no substantial difference between death from support withdrawal and death by active intervention (including the intervention of removing vital organs). This claim is controversial, and there have been two distinct challenges to their position. One objection focuses on the right of individuals to noninterference. The autonomous refusal of life support, whether by requesting the withholding or the withdrawing of life support, must be respected, lest physicians be liable for battery or assault. But competent patients cannot demand treatments, and thus, they cannot demand the removal of a vital organ when its removal is not clinically indicated. A second objection is based on the doctrine of double effect. This doctrine holds that an evil effect (e.g., death) can be morally tolerable if it is a side effect of an action undertaken with a good intention, if the evil effect is not a means to the good one, and if the harm is proportional to the good effect.[10] This is a widely held view first developed by Roman Catholic theologians but later adopted by many secular thinkers, the American Medical Association, the American courts, and (with qualifications) an important president's commission.[11] The mainstream of Western thinking relies on the doctrine of double effect or on other related arguments in order to assert the position that forgoing life support can be morally tolerable when the treatment is useless or gravely burdensome, considering the circumstances. By contrast, the removal of organs and the ensuing death cannot be considered a "side effect" but rather is a means to the good effect of benefiting those who receive the transplants. Hence, the mainstream of Western thinking has consistently rejected Miller and Truog's position that killing to procure organs is no different from withdrawing life support.[12] Even Miller and Truog, however, concede that such procurement not only is presently illegal but also is not likely to be legalized in the foreseeable future.[13] However, at least one study shows that this idea is gaining traction, at least theoretically, among the public at large.[14]

Candidates for a Concept of Death

As long as ethically and legally legitimate organ procurement for transplanting life-prolonging organs is so closely tied to death—that is, as long as we accept the dead donor rule—it becomes crucial to understand with clarity and precision what it means to be dead. But answering this question is not as simple as it might seem.

Four Concepts of Death

There are several plausible candidates for a concept of death. All are attempts to determine what is so significant to a human being that its loss constitutes the ultimate change in the moral and legal status of the individual. Here, we focus on four main concepts of death. First, the traditional religious and philosophical view in Western culture was that a human died at the time when the soul left the body. This separation of body and soul is difficult to verify scientifically and is best left to the religious traditions, which in some cases still focus on this soul-departure concept of death.

Traditional secular thinkers have held a second concept of death, one that focused on the cessation of the flow of the vital body fluids, blood and breath; thus, when the circulatory and respiratory functions cease irreversibly, the individual is dead. This view of the nature of the human being identifies the human essence with the flowing of fluids in the animal species. Variations on this view are still held by some, including those who oppose organ procurement before death and also some who are prepared to abandon the dead donor rule.

There are also two new candidates for a concept of death. One of these is that death occurs when there is a complete loss of the body's integrating capacities, which have, until the very recent discussion of the inclusivity of brain functions vis-à-vis death, been signified by the activity of the central nervous system. This third candidate for a concept of what it means to be dead has for the past half century been closely associated with what is popularly, if ambiguously, called "brain death." However, recently in the literature, some have begun to question the adequacy of this notion of death, claiming either that it is too inclusive, by including brain functions that are not critical, or that it is not inclusive enough, because it omits integrative functions that are not brain based. Some ask, Why must one identify the entire brain with death; is it not possible that we are really interested only in certain more important brain functions? For example, the now-standard definition of death based on brain function loss considers the presence of lower-brain reflexes, such as the gag reflex, as evidence of brain function. Therefore, an individual who has lost all brain functions except for the gag reflex would need to be classified as alive because he or she has not lost all functions of the entire brain. Because they consider someone with any brain function as alive, definitions based on the loss of all brain functions are now sometimes called "whole-brain-death" definitions. We explore these whole-brain definitions in the next chapter. Some critics, however, now insist that important integrative functions of the body—including circulation, excretion, and reproduction—can be present even in the absence of any brain functions. This has led some to revert to a definition of death that places critical importance on circulation, a view we explore in chapter 4.

Those who reject the idea that literally any brain function counts as evidence of a living human being believe that only certain more important brain functions should count. For example, human consciousness—the ability to think, reason, feel, experience, interact with others, and control body functions consciously—might be considered necessary. Because these functions are generally associated with the cerebral cortex, the anatomically and evolutionarily higher portion of the brain, this fourth view is sometimes called the "higher-brain-death" definition. In chapter 5 we sketch the arguments related to this higher-brain view. First, however, we need to clarify two issues that influence any definition of death, and then we can identify the public policy issues at stake in the definition-of-death debate.

Moral, Not Technical

The debate about the meaning of death involves a choice among these candidates for death and other variants we shall encounter in succeeding chapters. The committee we described in the introduction, the Harvard Ad Hoc Committee to Examine the Definition of Brain Death, was a committee at Harvard Medical School made up of physicians, lawyers, theologians, and social scientists. It established four operational criteria for what it called an irreversible coma, based on what was then taken to be very sound scientific evidence. These four criteria are (1) unreceptivity and unresponsivity, (2) no movements or breathing, (3) no reflexes, and (4) a flat EEG ("of great confirmatory value").[15]

What the committee did not do, however, and what it was not capable of doing, was establish that patients in an irreversible coma are "dead"—that is, that we should treat them as if they were no longer living human beings who possess the same moral rights and obligations as other living people. Although it may be the case that patients in an irreversible coma, according to the Harvard criteria, have shifted to that status where they are no longer to be considered living, the decision that they are "dead" cannot be derived from any amount of scientific investigation and demonstration of the brain's status. The choice among the many candidates for what is essential to the nature of the species, the loss of which, therefore, is to be called "death," is a philosophical or moral question, not a medical or scientific one.

Thus, in the definition-of-death debate we encounter a fundamental fact-value issue. There are two more or less separate questions at stake—one normative, the other scientific. The normative question is, What change in a human being is so fundamental that we can say the individual is no longer with us as a member of the human community bearing rights such as the right not to be killed? The answers involve some irreversible change—in the flowing of vital fluids (blood and breath), in the integration of the organism under the control of the brain, or perhaps in the dissociation of consciousness from organic (bodily) function. Choosing the point at which we should treat humans the way we treat dead people turns out to be a normative issue, not a scientific one. Expertise in neurology or cardiology does not prepare one to provide an answer. Any layperson can form an opinion.

Once we have answered the normative question, we can then move on to ask the scientific question, How do we know that some element critical for human status—the flowing of fluids, the integrative activity of the brain, or the capacity for consciousness—has been lost irreversibly? This second question should be largely the domain of medical science. Laypeople lack the expertise to play a direct role in providing an answer. The first question, however—that is, the normative question—is one that laypeople play a central role in answering. No amount of expertise in medical science can tell us whether fluid flow, integrative brain function, or capacity for consciousness is the normatively critical function for assigning the moral and legal status to a human as a living member of the human community.

The Irreversibility Problem

A second issue influences the definition of death. It arises no matter which definition of death one chooses: Must the function loss be irreversible, and if so, what does this mean? Most standard definitions of death include the requirement that the critical function loss, whatever that may be, must be irreversible. Thus, a mistake, potentially a serious mistake, is made if a patient who has suffered cardiac arrest and is then successfully resuscitated is described as having "died and been brought back to life." Other equally confusing and misleading terminology is sometimes used; for example, the patient may be said to have suffered "clinical death."

The Language of Death

If death is, by definition, irreversible, then these accounts of such occurrences as "clinical death" logically must be wrong. One cannot suffer "death" and be brought back to life. "Clinical death" is a meaningless term and is used erroneously if it is made a synonym for suffering cardiac arrest. At no time during an episode of cardiac arrest followed by a successful resuscitation that restores cardiac function was the patient ever dead.

There are very practical issues related to this linguistic point. When one dies, many important social and psychological events occur. One is obviously no longer covered by health insurance; life insurance, conversely, pays off to the beneficiary. One's spouse becomes a widow or widower and is free to remarry. The preparation for burial begins in a way that was not appropriate when the person's loved ones merely anticipated that death was imminent. For the purposes of transplants, one can, with proper authorization, remove vital organs.

It would be a disaster if one triggered any of these behaviors by calling someone dead if the patient's condition were reversible—if, say, cardiac arrest or a loss of brain function could be reversed.[16]

Legal versus Physiological Irreversibility

Assuming that dying is an irreversible event, some ambiguity nonetheless remains. In particular, how ought we to understand the moral and legal status of someone whose function loss could be reversed but will not be? This problem could arise, for example, if someone suffers cardiac arrest in a nursing home or small hospital that lacks the equipment to intervene to reverse the arrest. It might arise if the arrest could be reversed if a physician or someone trained in advanced lifesaving skills were on the scene, but no such person is around. Should we say that such a person is dead as long as the loss will not be reversed, even though it could be reversed if only the proper personnel or equipment were available, or should we wait until the loss could not be reversed under any circumstances?

There is an even more important variation on this problem. Should we call someone dead whose function loss could be reversed but will not be because that person (or that person's legally authorized surrogate) has refused life support using an advance directive or other mechanism to refuse consent to resuscitation? What if the patient's function loss could be reversed but will not be because a refusal of consent for cardiopulmonary resuscitation would make intervention illegal and presumably unethical?

If we say that such people are not really dead as long as they could be resuscitated (even though it would be illegal to do so), we face a serious issue in the routine clinical care of the terminally ill. Consider an elderly, terminally ill patient with metastatic cancer who has refused all further life support. This person will eventually suffer cardiac arrest. At such time, a physician on the scene could potentially restart the heart but obviously will not. Instead, the physician would plausibly note that the patient has died and pronounce the death to have occurred. The time of cardiac arrest would plausibly be listed as the time of death, not the time several minutes later when resuscitation would be physiologically impossible.

Some commentators have described this distinction as the difference between physiological irreversibility and legal or moral irreversibility. At the time of the arrest, or very soon thereafter, legal or moral irreversibility has occurred. It can be said with certainty that function loss is irreversible in the sense that we know functions will not resume. We say "very soon thereafter" because—as well shall see when we discuss organ procurement following circulatory arrest—we need to wait long enough to rule out a spontaneous restarting of the heart, what is called "autoresuscitation." We pronounce death in such cases even though, physiologically, a skilled medical professional could still likely restart the heart function. If this is what we mean by irreversibility, then death can be said to occur when function loss is legally or morally irreversible even though, physiologically, the process could possibly be reversed.

Some more conservative commentators, such as Don Marquis, have resisted this interpretation of irreversibility.[17] They believe that someone should not be called "dead" if the critical function loss could be reversed, even though it will not be. Those who see the concept of death in biological terms believe that organisms whose function could be restored should not be called dead even if the function is permanently lost.

Marquis and others are now sometimes explicating this situation by distinguishing between "permanent" and "irreversible" loss, where permanent has more or less the same meaning as "legally or morally irreversible." Because the laws defining death specify that death is an irreversible event, limiting the word "irreversible" to physiological irreversibility has important practical and legal significance. Loss that is merely permanent, but is not physiologically irreversible, is not death at all. Conversely, those willing to treat as dead those people who have lost function and will not have it restored (i.e., those who equate death with permanent loss) are more likely to use permanence and legal irreversibility interchangeably, thus making such loss consistent with definition-of-death statutes that ambiguously require "irreversibility" without specifying which kind.

Thus, unless we overturn the dead donor rule, an action that would require a major change in the law as well as revision of the cultural consensus, we may procure life-prolonging organs only from dead people. And now, for public policy purposes—including organ procurement—we therefore need to understand precisely what it means to say that someone is dead.

The Public Policy Question

The public policy discussion of how to define death began in earnest in the late 1960s, not long before surgeons were confronted by Bruce Tucker's case. Now, a half century later, we are still unclear about exactly what it means to be dead. The 1960s debate began in the context of a world that had in the previous decade seen the first successful transplantation of an organ from one human being to another. By 1967 we had seen the first transplantation of a human heart. It cannot be denied that this sudden infatuation with the usefulness of human organs was the stimulus for the intense debate about the real meaning of death. What many thought would be a rather short-lived debate, resolved by the combined wisdom of the health professionals and the nonscientists on the Harvard Ad Hoc Committee to Examine the Definition of Brain Death, has lingered as an intractable morass of conflicting technical, legal, conceptual, and moral arguments. Much of this confusion can be avoided, however, by focusing exclusively on the public policy dimensions of the debate about when death occurs.

Focusing on public policy means avoiding a full linguistic analysis of the term "death." Although that may be an important philosophical project, and many have undertaken it, such an analysis would be of only indirect importance for public policy questions.[18] Likewise, we need not provide a detailed theological account of the meaning of death. Such studies are numerous, but they are not of immediate concern for the formation of secular public policy.[19] Nor are we concerned about the ontological question of when an entity ceases to be human. Some philosophers have tried to turn the definition-of-death debate into such a deep philosophical exploration.[20] Most significantly, it is not necessary to give a scientific description of the biological events in the brain at the time of death. Of course, this description is of crucial importance for the science of neurology, and a vast literature is available giving such an account.[21] But the scientific, biological, and neurological descriptions of precisely what takes place in the human body at the point of death are not a matter that need directly concern makers of public policy.

Instead, what we are interested in is the answer to one key public policy question: When should we begin treating an individual the way we treat the newly dead? Is it possible to identify a point in the course of human events at which a new set of social behaviors becomes appropriate—at which, because we say the individual has died, we may justifiably begin to treat him or her in a way that was not previously appropriate, morally or legally? In short, what we are interested in is a social system of *death behaviors*.

Social and cultural changes take place when we label someone as dead. Perhaps some medical treatments may be stopped when an individual is considered dead that would not be stopped if the individual were alive—even if the living individual were terminally ill. This, of course, does not imply that there are treatments that should not be stopped at other times, either before or after the moment when we label someone as dead. Many treatments are stopped before death for technical reasons. Other treatments, including some that prolong life, may justifiably be stopped before death because they are no longer appropriate, because they either no longer serve a useful purpose or are too burdensome. In other cases, if the newly dead body is to be used for research, education, or transplant purposes, it is possible to continue certain interventions even after death has been declared. Many have held that this is morally acceptable.[22] However, it appears that, at least traditionally, some treatments have been stopped when and only when we have decided that it is time to treat the individual as dead.

Other behaviors, some of which were described earlier in this chapter, also have traditionally taken place at the time we consider the individual dead—behaviors such as mourning in a pattern that is not appropriate for mere anticipatory grief, beginning the process that will lead to reading the person's will, burying or otherwise disposing of what we now take to be the person's "mortal remains," and assuming the role of widowhood or widowerhood.[23] Perhaps of most immediate relevance to the concern that generated the definition-of-death debate, we change the procedures and justifications for obtaining organs from the body. Assuming we continue to accept the dead donor rule, before death, organs can be removed only in the interests of the individual, or perhaps in procurements that are not expected to lead to the individual's death, with the consent of the individual or his or her legal guardian.[24] At the moment we decide to treat someone as dead, an entirely different set of procedures is called for.

For the United States the procedures were originally designated in the Uniform Anatomical Gift Act, which was drawn up in 1968 and more recently has been refined in several revisions.[25] At this point, if one has agreed while alive to donate organs after one has died, the organs may be removed according to the terms of the donation without further consideration of the interest of the former individual or the wishes of his or her family members. If the deceased has not expressed his or her wishes to donate but has also not expressed opposition to donation, the next of kin or other legitimate guardian in possession of the body assumes both the right and the responsibility for the disposal of the remains and may donate the organs.

It is clear that at least in Anglo-American law, the person with such a responsibility cannot merely dispose of the body capriciously in any way he or she sees fit but bears a responsibility to treat the new corpse with respect and dignity.[26] This, however, has been taken both in law and in morality as permitting the donation of body parts by the one with this responsibility, except when an explicit objection was expressed by the now deceased during his or her life.

In short, traditionally there has been a radical shift in moral, social, and political standing when someone has been labeled as dead. Until the 1960s there was not a great deal of controversy over exactly when such a label should be applied. There were deviant philosophical and theological positions and substantial concern about the erroneous labeling of someone as dead, but there was very little real controversy about what it meant to be dead in this public policy sense.

Now, for the first time, there are matters of real public policy significance in deciding precisely what we mean when we label someone dead. In an earlier day all the socially significant death-related behaviors were generated at the time of death pronouncement. Very little was at stake if we were not precise in sorting out the various indicators of the time when this behavior was appropriate. Virtually all the plausible events related to death occurred in rapid succession, and none of the behaviors was really contingent on having any greater precision.

But matters have changed in two important ways. First, several technologies have greatly extended our capacity to prolong the dying process, making it possible to identify several different events that could be potential indicators of what we should take to be the death of the individual as a whole, and have separated these events dramatically in time. Second, the usefulness of human organs and tissues for transplantation, research, and education makes precision morally imperative. In an earlier day the most that was at stake was that an individual could for a few seconds be falsely treated as alive when in fact he or she should have been treated as dead, or vice versa. Of course, it is crucial, out of our sense of respect for persons, that we not confuse living individuals with their corpses, so in theory it has always been important that we be clear about whether someone is dead or alive. Yet, traditionally, the very short time frame for the entire series of events meant that very little was at stake as a matter of public policy. We could pronounce death on the basis of the rapid succession of an inevitably linked series of bodily events—heart stoppage, stoppage of respiration, or the death of the brain—without determining exactly which event was critical.

As we extend the length of time over which these events can occur, which in turn permits much more precision in identifying what in the human body signifies that it should be treated as dead, we must ask the question, Can we continue to identify a single, definable point when all the social behaviors associated with death should begin? It may turn out that as the dying process is extended, all these behaviors will find their own niches and that it really will cease to be important to label someone as dead at a precise moment in time. This has been called "disaggregation."[27] Life-sustaining treatment could then be stopped at one moment, mourning begun at another, and life insurance payoffs and funeral preparations made or started at still others. In this new context, organ procurement could take place at its own special moment, independent of exactly when death is pronounced. If so, death itself, and also dying, could begin to be viewed as a process.[28]

However, it seems likely that this will not happen. Rather, we may want to continue to link many of these social events, so we shall continue to say that there is a moment when it becomes appropriate to begin the entire series of death behaviors—or at least many of them. If so, then the death of an individual as a whole will continue to be viewed as a single event, rather than as a process.[29] There are several plausible candidates for this critical point when we can say that the individual as a whole has died—including the time when circulatory function ceases, the time when all brain functions cease, and the time when certain important brain functions, such as mental function, cease.

The question is therefore not precisely the same as the one the philosopher asks when he or she explores the end point of personhood or personal identity.[30] Analyses of the concept of personhood or personal identity suggest that there may be an identifiable end point at which we should stop thinking of a human organism as a *person*. This analysis by itself, however, never tells us whether it is morally appropriate to begin treating that human the way we have traditionally treated the dead, unless personhood is simply defined with reference to death behavior, which it often is not.

Under some formulations, such as those of Michael Green and Daniel Wikler, it is conceptually possible to talk about a living individual in cases where the person no longer exists.[31] (This would be true, for example, if we said that living humans were persons only when they possessed self-awareness or the ability to distinguish themselves from others.[32]) Some human individuals could then be alive but not considered persons. Logically, we would then be pressed to the moral and policy question of whether these living bodies that are no longer persons are to be treated differently from the way we are used to treating living persons.

Fortunately, for matters of public policy, if not for philosophical analysis, we need not take up the question of personhood or personal identity but can directly confront the question of whether we can identify a point when this series of death behaviors is appropriate. In this way death comes to mean, for public policy purposes, nothing more than the condition of some group of human beings for whom death behavior is appropriate. Can we identify this point? If we can, then, for purposes of law and public policy, we shall label this point as the moment of death. The laws reformulating the definition of death do not go so far as to say that they are defining death for all purposes—theological, philosophical, and personal. Some explicitly limit the scope, saying that the law defines death "for all *legal* purposes."

We now recognize that this point at which a group of death behaviors is considered appropriate may not exactly match the end point of biological life, or even the point at which the integrated functioning of an organism ceases. Thus, the word "death" may have come to have more than one meaning. The end point of the organism's integrated functioning may not be the same as the point when society calls the individual dead for legal and public policy purposes. If the term "death" takes on multiple meanings, it will have many similarities to the word "person."

The term "person" now has both nonmoral and moral meanings. The nonmoral meaning equates persons with self-aware beings; the moral meaning equates persons with beings who are the bearers of human rights (e.g., the right not to be killed). Thus, conservatives on abortion can argue for a constitutional amendment specifying that humans are "persons" from the moment of conception, without implying that the preembryo is a self-aware being. By this same bit of linguistic ambiguity, it is possible that some may be dead for public policy purposes even though biological functions remain.

In the past decade, as we have discovered the increasing complexity of the concept of death, we have been facing a linguistic choice. As it becomes increasingly clear, for example, that individuals who have irreversibly lost all brain functions may nevertheless retain many biological functions that make the body perform as an integrated whole, we could insist that the word "death" retain its traditional biological meaning and claim that those with dead brains may not necessarily be dead people. In retrospect that may have been the simpler use of terms. However, in the decades since the original proposal for brain-based concepts of death, laws and public discourse have established the pattern of also using the term "death" to refer to those beings who should be treated the way we treat the dead. The term "death," then, like the term "person," has taken on a second meaning—a moral as well as a biological meaning. One approach is to ask, for public policy purposes, which beings should be treated the way we treat dead people, and call those people "dead." That is the current usage. Laws in all US jurisdictions (and in most other countries of the world) affirm that individuals who have irreversibly lost certain functions shall be treated as dead, even though some biological functions, such as circulation, remain. The question for the following chapters is, When, for public policy purposes, should we treat human beings the way we treat the dead—when should we call them "dead" in this second sense of the term?

In the next three chapters, omitting the religious concept involving the departure of the soul, we examine the three major answers (or groups of answers) to this question. We look first at what we call the whole-brain answers; then at the circulatory, or somatic, answers; and finally at the higher-brain answers.

Notes

1. Tucker v. Lower, No. 2831 (Richmond, VA, L & Eq. Ct., May 23, 1972); Frederick RS II, "Medical jurisprudence: determining the time of death of the heart transplant donor," *North Carolina Law Review* 1972;51(6):172–184.

2. "'Brain death' held proof of demise in Va. jury decision," *Internal Medicine News*, July 1, 1992, 19.

3. "Virginia jury rules that death occurs when brain dies," *New York Times*, May 27, 1972.

4. Harvard Medical School, "A definition of irreversible coma: report of the Ad Hoc Committee of the Harvard Medical School to Examine the Definition of Brain Death," *JAMA* 1968;205(6):337–340.

5. Robertson JA, "Relaxing the death standard for organ donation in pediatric situations," in *Organ Substitution Technology: Ethical, Legal, and Public Policy Issues*, ed. Mathieu D (Boulder, CO: Westview Press, 1988), 69–76; Fost N, "Organs from anencephalic infants: an idea whose time has not yet come," *Hastings Center Report* 1988;18(5):5–10.

6. On the morality of intentional killings, see Rachels J, "Active and passive euthanasia," *New England Journal of Medicine* 1975; 292(2):78–80; Quill T, *Death and Dignity: Making Choices and Taking Charge* (New York: W. W. Norton, 1993); Beauchamp TL, *Intending Death: The Ethics of Assisted Suicide and Euthanasia* (Upper Saddle River, NJ: Prentice Hall, 1996); Battin MP, *Ending Life: Ethics and the Way We Die* (New York: Oxford University Press, 2005). On the legalization of intentional killings, see Quill et al. v. Vacco et al., Docket No. 95–7028, US Court of Appeals for the Second Circuit; Compassion in Dying v. Washington, No. 94–35534 D.C. No. CV-94-119-BJR, US Court of Appeals for the Ninth Circuit.

7. On the positions of professional groups, see American Medical Association, Council on Ethical and Judicial Affairs, *AMA's Code of Ethics*, opinion 2.21, issued June 1994, updated June 1996, www.ama-assn.org/ama/pub/physician-resources/medical-ethics/code-medical-ethics/opinion221.page?. On the positions of academics, see Foot P, "Active euthanasia with parental consent," *Hastings Center Report* 1979;9(5):20–21; Gaylin W, Kass L, Pellegrino E, Siegler M, "Doctors must not kill," *JAMA* 1988;259(14):2139–2140; Pellegrino ED,

"Doctors must not kill," in *Euthanasia: The Good Patient*, ed. Misbin RI (Frederick, MD: University Publishing Group, 1992), 27–42; Kamisar Y, "Are laws against assisted suicide unconstitutional?" *Hastings Center Report* 1993;23(3):32–41. On the positions of religious bodies, see US Conference of Catholic Bishops, *Ethical and Religious Directives for Catholic Health Care Services*, 5th ed. (Washington, DC: US Catholic Conference, 2009), www.usccb.org/issues-and-action /human-life-and-dignity/health-care/upload/Ethical-Religious -Directives-Catholic-Health-Care-Services-fifth-edition-2009.pdf.

8. Fost N, "The unimportance of death," in *The Definition of Death: Contemporary Controversies*, ed. Youngner SJ, Arnold RM, Schapiro R (Baltimore: Johns Hopkins University Press, 1999), 172–174; Koppelman ER, "The dead donor rule and the concept of death: severing the ties that bind them," *American Journal of Bioethics* 2003;3(1):1–9; Rodríguez-Arias D, Smith MJ, Lazar NM, "Donation after circulatory death: burying the dead donor rule," *American Journal of Bioethics* 2011;11(8):36–43.

9. Truog RD, Miller FG, "The dead donor rule and organ transplantation," *New England Journal of Medicine* 2008;359(7):674–675; Miller FG, Truog RD, *Death, Dying, and Organ Transplantation* (New York: Oxford University Press, 2012); Miller FG, Truog RD, Brock DW, "The dead donor rule: can it withstand critical scrutiny?" *Journal of Medicine and Philosophy* 2010;35(3):299–312.

10. McCormick RA, Ramsey P, eds., *Doing Evil to Achieve Good: Moral Choice in Conflict Situations* (Chicago: Loyola University Press, 1978); Graber GC, "Some questions about double effect," *Ethics in Science and Medicine* 1979;6(1):65–84; Marquis DB, "Four versions of double effect," *Journal of Medicine and Philosophy* 1991;16(5):515–544; Pellegrino ED, "Intending to kill and the principle of double effect," in *Ethical Issues in Death and Dying*, 2nd ed., ed. Beauchamp TL, Veatch RM (Englewood Cliffs, NJ: Prentice Hall, 1995), 240–242.

11. President's Commission for the Study of Ethical Problems in Medicine and Biomedical and Behavioral Research, *Deciding to Forgo Life-Sustaining Treatment: Ethical, Medical, and Legal Issues in Treatment Decisions* (Washington, DC: US Government Printing Office, 1983), 80–82.

12. On Western thinking, see Veatch RM, "The dead donor rule: true by definition," *American Journal of Bioethics* 2003;3(1):10–11; McCartney JJ, "The theoretical and practical importance of the dead donor rule," *American Journal of Bioethics* 2003;3(1):15–16; Vernez SL,

Magnus D, "Can the dead donor rule be resuscitated?" *American Journal of Bioethics* 2011;11(8):1; Chen YY, Ko WJ, "Further deliberating burying the dead donor rule in donation after circulatory death," *American Journal of Bioethics* 2011;11(8):58–59. For Miller and Truog's position, see Miller and Truog, *Death, Dying*, 14–18.

13. Miller and Truog, *Death, Dying*, 151.

14. Nair-Collins M, Green SR, Sutin AR, "Abandoning the dead donor rule? a national survey of public views on death and organ donation," *Journal of Medical Ethics* 2015;41(4):297–302.

15. Harvard Medical School, "Definition of irreversible coma."

16. There exists in the philosophical literature pertaining to the definition of death a minority view holding that death is indeed a reversible event and that those who suffer a cardiac arrest and are resuscitated are properly said to have died and been brought back to life. This usage is overwhelmingly rejected, however, in favor of insisting that if the arrest is reversed, death never occurred, only a cardiac arrest that would have led to death had not the arrest been reversed. See Cole DJ, "The reversibility of death," *Journal of Medical Ethics* 1992;18(1):26–30; Cole D, "Statutory definitions of death and the management of terminally ill patients who may become organ donors after death," *Kennedy Institute of Ethics Journal* 1993;3(2):145–155. Cf. Lamb D, "Reversibility and death: a reply to David Cole," *Journal of Medical Ethics* 1992;18(1):31–33; Tomlinson T, "The irreversibility of death: reply to Cole," *Kennedy Institute of Ethics Journal* 1993;3(2):157–165.

17. Marquis D, "Are DCD donors dead?" *Hastings Center Report* 2010;40(3):24–31. Even some commentators who hold very liberal views regarding organ procurement have taken the position that mere permanent function loss should not count as death. See Miller and Truog, *Death, Dying*, 106–107.

18. Becker LC, "Human being: the boundaries of the concept," *Philosophy and Public Affairs* 1975;4(4):334–359; Cole, "Reversibility of death"; Green MB, Wikler D, "Brain death and personal identity," *Philosophy and Public Affairs* 1980;9(2):105–133; Lamb, "Reversibility and death"; Mayo D, Wikler D, "Euthanasia and the transition from life to death," in *Medical Responsibility: Paternalism, Informed Consent, and Euthanasia*, ed. Robinson W, Pritchard MS (Clifton, NJ: Humane Press, 1979); Veatch RM, *Death, Dying, and the Biological Revolution*, rev. ed. (New Haven, CT: Yale University Press, 1989); Veatch RM, "The definition of death: unresolved controversies," in *Pediatric Brain Death and Organ/Tissue Retrieval*, ed. Kaufman HH (New York: Plenum, 1989),

207–218; Wikler D, Weisbard AJ, "Appropriate confusion over 'brain death,'" *JAMA* 1989;261(15):2246; Youngner SJ, Landefeld CS, Coulton CJ, Juknialis BW, Leary M, "'Brain death' and organ retrieval," *JAMA* 1989;261(15):2205–2210; Bonelli RM, Prat EH, Bonelli J, "Philosophical considerations on brain death and the concept of the organism as a whole," *Psychiatria Danubina* 2009;21(1):3–8; Degrazia D, "The definition of death," *Stanford Encyclopedia of Philosophy*, October 26, 2007, updated August 25, 2011, http://plato.stanford.edu/entries/death-definition/; Kagan S, *Death* (New Haven, CT: Yale University Press, 2012).

19. Bleich JD, "Neurological criteria of death and time-of-death status," in *Jewish Bioethics*, ed. Bleich JD, Rosner F (New York: Sanhedrin Press, 1979), 303–316; Bleich JD, "Of cerebral, respiratory, and cardiac death," *Tradition: A Journal of Orthodox Jewish Thought* 1989;24(3):44–66; Fletcher J, "Our shameful waste of human tissue," in *Updating Life and Death*, ed. Cutler DR (Boston: Beacon Press, 1969), 1–27; Haring B, *Medical Ethics* (Notre Dame, IN: Fides Press, 1973); Hauerwas S, "Religious concepts of brain death and associated problems," in *Brain Death: Interrelated Medical and Social Issues*, ed. Korein J (New York: New York Academy of Sciences, 1978), 329–338; Pope Pius XII, "The prolongation of life: an address of Pope Pius XII to an international congress of anesthesiologists," *The Pope Speaks* 1958;4:393–398; Ramsey P, *The Patient as Person* (New Haven, CT: Yale University Press, 1970), 59–164.

20. Green, Wikler, "Brain death," 105–133; cf. Gervais KG, *Redefining Death* (New Haven, CT: Yale University Press, 1986).

21. Ashwal S, Schneider S, "Brain death in children, part I," *Pediatric Neurology* 1987;3(1):5–11; Ashwal S, Schneider S, "Brain death in children, part II," *Pediatric Neurology* 1987;3(2):69–78; Black PM, "Brain death (first of 2 parts)," *New England Journal of Medicine* 1978;299(7):338–344; Black PM, "Brain death (second of 2 parts)," *New England Journal of Medicine* 1978;299(8):393–401; "An appraisal of the criteria of cerebral death: a summary statement. A collaborative study," *JAMA* 1977;237(10):982–986; Cranford RE, Beresford R, Caronna JJ, Conomy JP, Hardy PM, "Uniform Brain Death Act," *Neurology* 1979;29(3):417–418; Harvard Medical School, "Definition of irreversible coma"; O'Brien MD, "Criteria for diagnosing brain stem death," *British Medical Journal* 1990;301(6743):108–109; "Report of the medical consultants on the diagnosis of death to the President's Commission for the Study of Ethical Problems in Medicine and Biomedical

and Behavioral Research," in *Defining Death: Medical, Legal and Ethical Issues in the Definition of Death*, ed. President's Commission for the Study of Ethical Problems in Medicine and Biomedical and Behavioral Research (Washington, DC: US Government Printing Office, 1981), 159–166; Shewmon DA, "Commentary on guidelines for the determination of brain death in children," *Annals of Neurology* 1988;24(6):789–791; Special Task Force for the Determination of Brain Death in Children, "Guidelines for the determination of brain death in children," *Pediatrics* 1987;80(2):298–300; Nakagawa TA, Ashwal S, Mathur M, Mysore M; Society of Critical Care Medicine, Section on Critical Care and Section of Neurology of the American Academy of Pediatrics, and the Child Neurology Society, "Clinical report—guidelines for the determination of brain death in infants and children: an update of the 1987 task force recommendations," *Pediatrics* 2011;128(3):e720–e740; Wijdicks EFM, Varelas PN, Gronseth GS, Greer DM, "Evidence-based guideline update: determining brain death in adults report of the Quality Standards Subcommittee of the American Academy of Neurology," *Neurology* 2010;74:1911–1918; Shemie SD, Hornby L, Baker A, et al.; International Guidelines for Determination of Death, Phase 1 Participants in collaboration with the World Health Organization, "International guideline development for the determination of death," *Intensive Care Medicine* 2014;40(6):788–797; Wijdicks EF, "Brain death guidelines explained," *Seminars in Neurology* 2015;35(2):105–115.

22. Haring, *Medical Ethics*; Ramsey, *Patient as Person*, 59–164.

23. Fulton R, Fulton J, "Anticipatory grief: a psychosocial aspect of terminal care," in *Psychosocial Aspects of Terminal Care*, ed. Schoenberg B, Carr AC, Peretz D, Kutscher AH (New York: Columbia University Press, 1972), 227–242.

24. Fellner CH, "Selection of living kidney donors and the problem of informed consent," *Seminars in Psychiatry* 1971;3(1):70–85; Mahoney J, "Ethical aspects of donor consent in transplantation," *Journal of Medical Ethics* 1975;1(2):67–70; Robertson JA, "Organ donations by incompetents and the substituted judgment doctrine," *Columbia Law Review* 1976;76(1):48–78; Simmons RG, Fulton J, "Ethical issues in kidney transplantation," *Omega* 1971;2(3):179–190.

25. National Conference of Commissioners on Uniform State Laws (NCCUSL), *Uniform Anatomical Gift Act* (Chicago: NCCUSL, 1968); NCCUSL, *Uniform Anatomical Gift Act (1987)* (Chicago: NCCUSL, 1987); NCCUSL, *Revised Uniform Anatomical Gift Act* (Chicago: NCCUSL, 2006).

26. May WF, "Attitudes toward the newly dead," *Hastings Center Studies* 1973;1(1):3–13.

27. Halevy A, Brody B, "Brain death: reconciling definitions, criteria, and tests," *Annals of Internal Medicine* 1993;119(6):519–525; Truog RD, "Is it time to abandon brain death?" *Hastings Center Report* 1997;27(1):29–37. See also Veatch RM, "The death of whole-brain death: the plague of the disaggregators, somaticists, and mentalists," *Journal of Medicine and Philosophy* 2005;30(4):353–378.

28. Morison R, "Death: process or event?" *Science* 1971;173(3998): 694–698.

29. Kass L, "Death as an event: a commentary on Robert Morison," *Science* 1971;173(3998):698–702.

30. Tooley M, "Decisions to terminate life and the concept of person," in *Ethical Issues Relating to Life and Death*, ed. Ladd J (New York: Oxford University Press, 1979), 62–93.

31. Green, Wikler, "Brain death."

32. One of us has argued this claim; see Veatch, "Dead donor rule."

3

The Whole-Brain Concept of Death

The concept of death that emerged in the second half of the twentieth century, the concept closely connected to the procurement of organs for transplant, is often simply referred to as brain death. It holds that an individual has died (and should be treated the way we treat dead people) when there is an irreversible loss of all functions of the entire brain. Those proposing such a concept make clear that it is all functions of the brain—including the brain stem—that must be lost, and they must be lost irreversibly. Because it is the functions of the entire brain that must be lost, sometimes this is referred to as the whole-brain concept of death.

Unfortunately, the term "brain death" has emerged in the debate over the definition of death. This is unfortunate in part because we are not interested in the death of brains; we are interested in the death of organisms as integrated entities subject to particular kinds of public behavior and control. The term "brain death" is systematically ambiguous. It has two potential meanings. The first is not controversial; it simply means the destruction of the brain, leaving open the question of whether people with destroyed brains should be treated as dead people (more precisely, as "dead former persons"). It is better to substitute the phrase "destruction of the brain" for brain death in this sense. It makes clear that we are referring only to the complete biological collapse of the organ or organs we call the brain. Exactly how that is measured is largely a neurological question.

Confusingly, "brain death" has also taken on a second, very different, and much more controversial meaning. It can also mean the death of the individual as a whole, based on the fact that the brain has died. The problem is illustrated in the original report of the Harvard Ad Hoc Committee, which became the most significant technical document in the early stages of the American debate.[1] The title of that 1968 document is "A Definition of Irreversible Coma." The article sets out to define "characteristics of irreversible coma" and produces a list of technical criteria that purport to predict that an individual is in a coma that is irreversible. The name of the committee, however, was the Harvard Ad Hoc Committee to Examine the Definition of Brain Death. The presumption apparently was that an irreversible coma and brain death were synonymous.

We now realize that this is not precisely true. An individual can apparently be in an irreversible coma and still not have a completely dead brain. To be even more precise, people can be either in an irreversible coma or in a persistent or permanent vegetative state (PVS) and still not have a completely dead brain. PVS is further differentiated from an irreversible coma in that those in an irreversible coma are in a perpetual sleep-like state, whereas those in PVS go through sleep-wake cycles and may appear to be alert, even though, by definition, they have no conscious experience. Some famous cases of patients in PVS were Karen Quinlan and Terri Schiavo. We now know that neither an irreversible coma nor PVS involves complete loss of all brain functions, even though they are permanent states of unconsciousness.

In any case the title of the report and the name of the committee, taken in the context of what the committee did, imply that the committee's objective was to describe the empirical measures of a destroyed brain. The opening sentence of the report, however, says, "Our primary purpose is to define irreversible coma as a new criterion for death." The report does not claim to define the destruction (death) of the brain, but death simpliciter, whereby everyone, including the committee members, meant the death of the individual for purposes of death behaviors, clinical practice, and public policy—including, of course, the procurement of life-prolonging organs in a way consistent with the dead donor rule. Yet the report contains no argument that the destruction of the brain (measured by the characteristics of an irreversible coma) should be taken as a justification for treating the individual as a whole as dead. The members of the committee and many others believed that this should be so, possibly with good reason, but the reasons were not stated.

Because the term "brain death" has these two radically different meanings, there is often confusion in public and professional discussions of the issues related to it. For instance, neurologists can claim that they have real expertise on brain death, meaning, of course, expertise in measuring the destruction of the brain. Others claim, however, that brain death is exclusively a matter for public policy consideration, meaning that the question of whether we should treat an individual as dead because the brain tissue is dead is outside the scope of neurological expertise. A far better course would be to abandon that language entirely, substituting precise and explicit language that either refers to the destruction of the brain or to the death of the individual as a whole based on brain criteria.

Debate over the past fifty years between those who consider death a matter of brain function and those who more traditionally consider death a matter of heart and lung (or circulation) function has created a situation whereby defenders of the neurological concepts of death have not been forced to be particularly precise in defining terms. The seemingly endless prolongation of cellular and organ functioning (in what can be appropriately called human corpses) has been brought about by new death-assaulting technologies, giving rise to a new and inhuman form of existence. Although the potential use of human organs for therapeutic transplantation should never justify the adoption of a new understanding of what is essentially significant to human life and death, the morally legitimate procurement of organs may require a philosophically responsible clarification of an imprecise use of these terms, which were adequate only in a time when little that was morally critical was at stake. These developments have led to an infatuation with neurologically oriented concepts, which have made the more traditional heart-and-lung definition of death appear inadequate and outmoded. The thesis of this chapter, however, is that the time has come when crude formulations of the so-called brain definition of death can no longer be tolerated.

Holders of the whole-brain-oriented concept of death would probably grant that the only practical problem with the more traditional concept, which focuses on the heart and lungs, is that it will on special occasions produce false positive tests for human life. In these rare cases individuals who should be considered dead are labeled alive because their heart and lung functions continue, even though brain function may have permanently and irreversibly ceased. Traditional moralists, however—or at least those who tend to hold a more rigorous, life-preserving position regarding moral obligations to an individual human being—prefer to err on the side of the morally safer course. Thus, Hans Jonas, one of the key players in the early definition-of-death debate, argued that unless one can be certain of the philosophical (technical uncertainty is not being considered here) foundations of the more limited brain-oriented concept, one should opt for the false positive judgment of continuing life rather than running the moral risk of a false pronouncement of death.[2]

The risk, then, is that of considering individuals with no brain function to be dead when in fact they are alive. Those who hold the brain-oriented concept of death have apparently satisfied themselves that there is no significant risk of this mistake being made.

The Case for the Whole-Brain Concept

In chapter 2 we introduced the distinction between the concept of death, which raises philosophical and normative questions, and the scientific criteria for death, the tests for the loss of what is so significant about human life that its loss constitutes death. The significance of this distinction can be seen if one begins with a completely formal definition of death: Death is the irreversible loss of that which is essentially significant to its nature.

Such a formal definition of death can be given substantive content only through further philosophical analysis. It is necessary to reach some understanding about what is essentially significant to the nature of the human. This cannot be determined by biological investigation but only by philosophical or theological reflection.

Although the Harvard Ad Hoc Committee did not offer any argument for a new brain-based concept of death, that project was nonetheless pursued over the following decade. The Research Group on Death and Dying of the Institute of Society, Ethics and the Life Sciences (now called the Hastings Center) took up the question in its 1972 review of the Harvard criteria.[3] This group, which included the chair of the Harvard Ad Hoc Committee, Henry Beecher, as well as a number of philosophically sophisticated thinkers such as Paul Ramsey, William May, and Daniel Callahan, recognized that there were problems in articulating a concept of death, problems not addressed by the Harvard committee. Its work pointed us in the direction of the consensus that was to emerge in the late twentieth century.

By 1981 a report titled *Defining Death* by the US President's Commission for the Study of Ethical Problems in Medicine and Biomedical and Behavioral Research clearly addressed the question.[4] It adopted a concept of death based on the irreversible loss of the body's integrating capacity: "Death is that moment at which the body's physiological system ceases to constitute an integrated whole. Even if life continues in individual cells or organs, life of the organism as a whole requires complex integration, and without the latter, a person cannot properly be regarded as alive."[5]

At about the same time, others were defining death as the "permanent cessation of functioning of the organism as a whole."[6] Often, a distinction was made between the "whole organism" and "the organism as a whole." The general belief was that the whole brain, not just the cerebrum, was the primary regulator of the functioning of the organism as a whole and that, therefore, the irreversible loss of all the functions of the entire brain constituted the death of the organism.

Thus, one candidate for the concept of death in humans is the irreversible loss of the body's capacity to function as an integrated whole. If we are speaking of the death of the organism as a whole— and not simply the death of isolated cells, organs, or organ systems— it at first seems plausible to consider the complex integrating capacity of an organism as that which is essential to it. If this is the case, then the loss of this integrating capacity could appropriately be equated with the organism's death. At the end of the twentieth century, it was accepted as common wisdom that the brain was the locus of this capacity. To be sure, the spinal cord and peripheral nerves are also important, but these do not really provide significant integration. The spinal reflexes at most provide a primitive and pale imitation of integrating function. The mysterious integrating capacity of the nervous system, which has fascinated humans and been conceptualized so influentially by Claude Bernard, is, by comparison, so much grander as to constitute the difference between a simple animal and the human organism.

It seemed reasonable from what we thought we knew about the brain to relate this concept of integrating capacity to the whole brain. If this is what is seen as essentially significant to the human, then the examination of the whole brain for signs of functioning is a plausible test of the death of the individual.

On the basis of these views, the President's Commission in 1981 endorsed the Uniform Determination of Death Act (UDDA) as containing the legal definition of death proposed by the American Bar Association, the American Medical Association, and the National Conference of Commissioners on Uniform State Laws. This act reads, "An individual who has sustained either (1) irreversible cessation of circulatory and respiratory functions; or (2) irreversible cessation of all functions of the entire brain, including the brain stem, is dead. A determination of death must be made in accordance with accepted medical standards."[7] These "accepted medical standards" have been debated over the years, giving rise to various sets of criteria that are sometimes referred to as criteria for death based on brain function loss.

Criteria for the Destruction of All Brain Functions

In the years since 1968, several sets of criteria have been proposed to measure the irreversible loss of all functions of the brain. In Europe it is common to rely on cerebral angiography.[8] In the United States the report of the Harvard Ad Hoc Committee provided the first widely accepted criteria set.

The Harvard Criteria, 1968

The Harvard report proposed four criteria:

1. unreceptivity and unresponsivity,
2. no movement or breathing,
3. no reflexes, and
4. a flat EEG.[9]

The fourth criterion, a flat EEG, was presented as being "of great confirmatory value" but not necessary. Presumably, if the first three criteria were met, then the EEG would need to be isoelectric, and an isoelectric EEG would necessarily require that the first three criteria were satisfied. The criteria set specifies that the EEG should be isoelectric when the gain is set at five microvolts per millimeter. This may be more controversial than it appears because it implies that very small amounts of electrical activity coming from the brain tissue can be ignored. Some activity could be from tissues surrounding the brain or from an artifact, but if even small amounts of electrical activity come from the brain itself, the tissue by implication is not really dead.

Tests based on these criteria were to be repeated at least twenty-four hours later with no change in findings. Two medical conditions, hypothermia and the presence of central nervous system depressants, had to be excluded.

The Minnesota Criteria, 1971

In 1971 a similar set of criteria was proposed by Mohandas and Chou, writing in the *Journal of Neurosurgery*.[10] They refined the reflex tests, excluded spinal reflexes,[11] and extended the period for the apnea testing from three to four minutes. They shortened the period for repeat testing to twelve hours and specifically rejected the need for an EEG.

National Institute of Neurological Diseases and Stroke, 1977

The National Institute of Neurological Diseases and Stroke formed a panel that developed further variations on the criteria set.[12] It added cardiovascular shock and remedial lesions to the list of exclusions and called for repeating tests six hours later. The EEG should show no activity greater than two microvolts per millimeter. The panel endorsed cerebral blood flow tests for confirmation.

Minnesota Medical Association Criteria, 1978

The Minnesota Medical Association endorsed a criteria set in 1978 that added intoxication as an exclusion criterion.[13] It accepted the three-minute apnea test and a twelve-hour period for repeat testing. It considered an EEG or angiography to be optional.

Medical Consultants to the President's Commission, 1981

The US President's Commission for the Study of Ethical Problems in Medicine and Biomedical and Behavioral Research established a group of medical consultants whose members presented their consensus criteria set as an appendix to the *Defining Death* report.[14] The consultants modified the Harvard criteria by adding neuromuscular blockade, cardiovascular shock, and metabolic disturbances to the exclusions, and they also excluded the use of the criteria in children below the age of five years. They extended the period of apnea testing to ten minutes and supported EEG or cerebral blood flow for confirmation. They proposed a more complex time interval for repeating the tests: six hours with confirmatory tests, twelve hours without, and twenty-four hours for anoxic brain damage. Furthermore, they required that the cause of coma be established.

American Academy of Pediatrics, 1987

The exclusion of children under five years old from the medical consultants' report to the President's Commission prompted the creation of a special task force of the American Academy of Pediatrics (AAP) to develop guidelines for the determination of brain death in children in 1987.[15] The AAP affirmed the definition of death and the requirements for its determination, noting that there were no unique legal issues for young children, only medical ones. Noting that the newborn is difficult to evaluate clinically after perinatal insults, the task force stated that the current criteria were valid in term newborns (greater than thirty-eight weeks' gestation) seven days after the neurologic insult. From seven days to two months, the task force recommended two examinations and EEGs separated by at least forty-eight hours. From two months to one year, the task force recommended two examinations and EEGs separated by at least twenty-four hours, although the second examination and EEG were not necessary if a concomitant cerebral radionuclide angiographic study demonstrated no visualization of cerebral arteries. For children older than one year, laboratory testing was not required when an irreversible cause existed, and the task force recommended an observation period of at least twelve hours. For some conditions, like hypoxic-ischemic encephalopathy, for which assessing the extent and reversibility of brain damage were difficult determinations, the task force recommended a more prolonged period of at least twenty-four hours of observation, which could be reduced if the EEG demonstrated electrocerebral silence or the cerebral radionuclide angiographic study did not visualize cerebral arteries. Other ancillary tests were being developed but were not yet ready for inclusion in the guidelines.

American Academy of Neurology, 1995

Responding to a perceived variability in the practice of diagnosis, in 1995 the American Academy of Neurology (AAN) published a set of practice parameters for diagnosing brain death.[16] Its criteria were similar to the 1981 criteria endorsed by the medical consultants to the President's Commission. It specified that the proximate cause of the brain pathology must be known and demonstrably irreversible. It also added electrolyte, acid-base, and endocrine disturbances to the list of medical conditions that must be excluded in order to make a determination of brain death, reduced the apnea test to eight minutes from the President's Commission's required ten minutes, and reduced the period for repeat testing to six hours.[17] It did not require confirmatory tests, such as an EEG and tests of cerebral blood flow, though it recommended such tests when other components of clinical testing could not be reliably performed or evaluated.

UK Academy of Medical Royal Colleges, 2008

In 2008 the Academy of Medical Royal Colleges in Great Britain published a report titled *A Code of Practice for the Diagnosis and Confirmation of Brain Death*.[18] Its criteria resembled the various American sets (a feature worth noting because, as we shall see later, Great Britain generally claims to be diagnosing only brain-stem function loss). It required that the clinicians exclude the presence of depressant drugs; potentially reversible circulatory, metabolic, and endocrine disturbances; and neuromuscular blocking agents as causes of unconsciousness, along with primary hypothermia. It required testing for reflexes, including pupillary light reflexes, oculovestibular reflexes, the corneal reflex, and the gag reflex. Apnea testing should last five minutes, and formal testing of brain-stem reflexes was usually carried out twice, twelve to twenty-four hours apart, by two experienced clinicians.

American Academy of Neurology, 2010

Addressing developments in technology and seeking research-based answers to outstanding questions, the AAN issued an update to its criteria in 2010.[19] The apnea test was changed from 8 minutes to 8–10 minutes. Although it had recommended a six-hour interval for retesting in 1995, in 2010 the AAN claimed that there was insufficient evidence to determine the minimally acceptable observation period, and it included no recommendation as to a retest interval. Ancillary tests, including EEG, nuclear scan, and cerebral angiogram, remained options whose use was suggested when there was uncertainty about other parts of the clinical evaluation.

American Academy of Pediatrics, Society of Critical Care Medicine, and Child Neurology Society, 2010

In 2010 the AAP Section on Critical Care, in conjunction with the Pediatric Section of the Society of Critical Care Medicine and the Child Neurology Society, revised and updated its guidelines for the establishment of brain death in children.[20] These guidelines held only for newborns (greater than thirty-seven weeks' gestational age) and older infants and children. The guidelines recommended a twenty-four-hour observation period for infants less than thirty days of age, and twelve hours for children between thirty days and eighteen years. As with the adult studies, ancillary studies were not necessary unless (1) the apnea test could not be completed safely owing to the condition of the patient, (2) uncertainty existed about the results of the neurologic examination, (3) a medication effect could be present, or (4) the inter-examination observation period was reduced. The guidelines stated that four-vessel cerebral angiography was the gold standard for determining the absence of cerebral blood flow but acknowledged that it was difficult to perform in infants and small children, might not be readily available, and required moving the patient to the angiography suite. EEG and the use of radionuclide cerebral blood flow determinations to document the absence of cerebral blood flow remained the most widely used methods to support the clinical diagnosis. Other ancillary studies—such as transcranial Doppler study, computed tomography (CT) angiography, CT perfusion using arterial spin labeling, nasopharyngeal somatosensory evoked potential studies, magnetic resonance imaging (MRI), magnetic resonance angiography (MRA), and perfusion MRI—had not been studied sufficiently nor validated in pediatrics at that time.

The Fact-Value Distinction Revisited

These criteria sets represent the consensus of medical experts on diagnostic criteria that identify brains that have irreversibly ceased to function. Recalling the distinction between scientific questions of the measurement of brain function and the more policy-oriented question of when someone should be treated as dead, almost everyone would recognize these criteria sets as scientific. They purport to be the best determiners of when a brain has irreversibly lost all its functions. (We shall see in the case of Jahi McMath later in this chapter and again in chapter 4 that, in fact, certain brain functions—such as neurohormonal regulation and some electrical evoked potentials—may remain, even though the criteria represented in these tests are met.) Although it is true that these criteria are grounded in neurological science, in them we discern some messy overlap between facts and value judgments.

Is the choice of criteria really a scientific question? In addition to the brain functions that are known to be compatible with patients who satisfy these criteria sets, some other assumptions are made that require normative judgments. For example, Henry Beecher was aware that some neurological integrative functions occurred in the spinal cord. These spinal reflexes are not greatly different from simple brain-stem reflexes and were included in the original Harvard Ad Hoc Committee report, but by 1971 Beecher felt comfortable excluding spinal cord reflexes as insignificant.[21] Another example in which value judgments impinge on statements of science is the different lengths of time for apnea testing in the different criteria sets: the Harvard criteria (1968), 3 minutes; University of Minnesota (1971), 4 minutes; National Institute of Neurological Diseases and Stroke (1977), 15 minutes; Minnesota Medical Association (1978), 3 minutes; President's Commission (1981), 10 minutes; AAN (1995), 8 minutes; and AAN (2010), 8–10 minutes. This variation is, at least in part, a function of how certain the various criteria set writers wanted to be.

Some of this variation may represent different understandings of scientific knowledge, but more may be at stake. The influence of normative judgments on the apparently scientific criteria sets is most clearly revealed in the choice of the time period over which tests should be repeated. Although published guidelines have been available for over forty years and have been revised as new evidence is discovered, the current data show that there is wide variability in the determination of death in both pediatric patients and adults.[22]

Consider that different criteria sets propose repeating tests over different periods: Harvard, 24 hours; Minnesota Medical Association, 12 hours; National Institute of Neurological Diseases and Stroke, 6 hours; and President's Commission, six to twenty-four hours. The most recent AAN criteria set (2010) proposes no clear interval for repeat tests. Part of the difference is the result of new scientific knowledge that has accumulated over the years. As more experience is gained, greater certainty is plausible and the interval for repetition can be reduced. Part of the difference, however, is a function of attitudes about how the possibility of error should be handled.

Two types of error are possible: Someone might falsely diagnose the death of the brain or might erroneously conclude the brain is alive when it is dead. Falsely diagnosing the death of the brain would mean labeling someone as having a brain without function when, in fact, functions remained. That seems like a serious error. Nevertheless, every diagnosis and prognosis has some possibility of error. The report of the National Institute of Neurological Diseases and Stroke panel said, "rarely (1 percent of cases) . . . the original reader diagnosed ECS [electro-cerebral silence] and the review panel considered that biological activity was present. . . . This 99 percent accuracy seems adequate for basic criteria."[23] In other words, the members of the panel were willing to adopt criteria that called some people dead when they actually retained brain function 1 percent of the time on the basis of a review panel's judgment. They thought that error was tolerable.

It is reported anecdotally that patients pronounced dead by traditional cardiac criteria were pronounced erroneously as much as 5 percent of the time. When one realizes that the patients falsely pronounced were nevertheless very near death, some would consider the errors not necessarily critical.

People also worry about the other type of error one might make: falsely labeling someone as living when they are, in fact, dead. In the case of death based on brain criteria, one sometimes worries that patients with loss of all functions of the brain might be for a time considered still alive when they are not.

Choosing the length of time between repeated tests is, in part, related to which type of error is of greater concern. If one wanted absolute certainty that brain function would never return, one could insist on repeating tests endlessly, thereby never judging too quickly. Picking the length of time between repeated tests is not only a function of advancement in scientific knowledge; it is also an evaluative judgment about the relative concern about the two types of error. The more one is concerned about falsely pronouncing death, the longer interval one will want between repeat tests. The more one is concerned about calling people alive when they are dead, the shorter the interval for repeating the tests. The interval chosen reflects a balance between these two types of error.

It may be that something as technical as choosing the gain on the machinery used for the EEG raises similar fact-value issues. The higher the gain, the less likely one is to miss small electrical potentials. One must make value-based choices about how small a potential is too small to worry about. For example, some neurologists have suggested that small electrical potentials may come off real brain tissues (and not be artifact or electrical potentials off other body tissues) but be only cellular-level activity. If one believes that only supercellular brain activity counts as a sign of life, then one would be inclined to ignore mere cellular activity and therefore attempt to exclude electrical potentials so low that they indicate only cellular activity.

Problems with the Whole-Brain Definition

In the past few years, there have been a number of court cases in which families have challenged the whole-brain definition or whole-brain determination of death. Here we discuss the recent cases of Jahi McMath and Aden Hailu.

The Case of Jahi McMath

In December 2013 a twelve-year-old girl, Jahi McMath, suffered severe bleeding after surgery for sleep apnea at an Oakland hospital. The loss of blood caused brain anoxia that led to the permanent loss of all brain functions as measured by standard tests, a fact confirmed by three sets of physicians, including one from a court-ordered independent expert neurologist. The hospital staff proposed following the standard practice of declaring Jahi dead based on brain function loss, but her mother, Nailah Winkfield, disagreed. Winkfield and her attorney subsequently made two different claims in court about Jahi's case. First, Winkfield disagreed that her daughter's brain function was irreversibly lost.[24] This claim was repeated in an amended complaint filed in November 2015 before the Superior Court of the State of California for the County of Alameda.[25] Second, Winkfield argued that, even if her daughter's brain function had been lost, Jahi was not dead as long as circulation and respiration remained (even if the respiration was the result of ventilatory support).[26] This second claim will be discussed in the next chapter. For now we will focus on Winkfield's disagreement with the determination of whole-brain death.

On January 3, 2014, the court did finally permit the hospital staff to declare Jahi dead in accordance with California law.[27] It went on, however, to consider the additional question of whether the staff could stop ventilatory and other support. The court finally arranged for Jahi to be released to the medical examiner while she was still on a ventilator (which maintained her circulatory and respiratory functions).[28] The medical examiner then released Jahi's body to her mother with the ventilator still running, thus permitting the mother to transfer her to an undisclosed facility that was willing to provide medical support for her legally dead body, which the mother insisted should be considered still alive.[29] As of this writing, it has been over two years since these events. Jahi was moved to New Jersey, where she (or her respiring dead body if one accepts the California death pronouncement) was placed in a medical facility. She was eventually moved to a private residence, where she continues to have her respiratory and circulatory functions maintained. In some instances it is technically possible to maintain a body with a dead brain for months or even years.[30] In chapter 6 we take up the question of whether the law should permit those who object to the standard law basing death on brain criteria to opt for the traditional circulatory definition. We shall also take up the question of who should bear responsibility for the costs involved.

In addition to the family's rejection of the brain-based death pronouncement, in legal actions the lawyer for Jahi's mother asked the Alameda County Superior Court in November 2015 to vacate the death certificate, claiming that Jahi did not meet the standard criteria for pronouncing death on the basis of brain criteria.[31] The legal action includes two claims.

First, it claims that video evidence and in-person examination shows that Jahi is responding to verbal commands to move a hand or foot. If this were true, everyone would agree Jahi is not dead by brain criteria. At first review the video seems to provide such evidence, but the defenders of the death pronouncement remain skeptical. The most suspicious complain that perhaps the tape was edited. We do not know how long the tape had to run to capture a movement that seemed to follow Jahi's mother's request for the movement. The claim acknowledges that Jahi was only "intermittently responding intentionally to a verbal command." Since we know that even patients with dead brains (i.e., those who meet the standard criteria for death based on brain function loss) occasionally make spontaneous movements, it requires complex and subjective judgment for the court to determine if the reported movements are really voluntary.

If the court were to find that Jahi fails to meet the standard brain-based criteria for death because she has the capacity for voluntary response, the effect on clinical practice could be enormous. One possibility for the mistaken diagnosis of death would be that the teams of neurologists who originally performed the tests that indicated Jahi's brain was dead somehow erred. This seems quite unlikely because the tests were performed by three separate teams of clinicians with acknowledged competence. Assuming the original tests were performed properly, a decision that Jahi shows responsivity years later suggests that the tests (and particularly the interval between repeated tests) were inadequate to prove irreversibility. This would undercut the entire practice of pronouncing death using the standard criteria sets we have described.

Second, the legal action claims that Jahi showed evidence of sexual maturation and menstruation, which, it claims, can occur only with activity of the hypothalamus (a part of the brain located just above the brain stem that links the nervous system to the endocrine system via the pituitary gland). Defenders of the original pronouncement of death claim that Jahi clearly showed evidence of sexual maturation before her surgery and subsequent brain pathology and that there is no evidence these functions were not present earlier. Thus, a clinical issue is being raised, and the court will have to settle. More important, it is not clear whether hormonal secretions from the hypothalamus or pituitary should count as evidence of brain function in the first place. Over the past forty-five-plus years, none of the standard criteria sets for brain death have included tests for such functions. Wijdicks provides a pathophysiologic explanation to exclude these functions because the hypothalamus and pituitary gland are perfused from extracranial vessels.[32] Moreover, we have known for at least thirty-five years that certain brain functions (including cellular-level functions, auditory evoked potentials, and hormonal secretions) can be present in brains determined to be dead by standard criteria.[33] This seems, on its face, to contradict the claim that "all functions of the entire brain" must be absent for brain death to be declared. Defenders of the standard tests say that we have always ignored certain brain functions as "irrelevant."[34] Strict critics of the current standard tests point out that the law clearly requires ruling out "all functions" and makes no provision for excluding certain "trivial" ones.[35] If the court agrees with the family that hypothalamic function is present, it will have to determine whether we can continue to exclude such functions or whether we must revise the criteria sets to include tests of hypothalamic functions. Thus, the court can demand a major change in determination of brain death from what is currently required in the United States and internationally.[36] In the past the judiciary has been quite deferential to medical professionals in the determination of death. According to the UDDA, "A determination of death must be made in accordance with accepted medical standards."[37] In a review of cases involving brain death, Burkle and colleagues found that "all court rulings upheld the medical practice of death determination using neurologic criteria according to state law, irrespective of other elements of the rulings."[38] The issue here is whether the public should accept the judgment of the medical profession about whether to exclude hormonal function and limit tests to neurological activity.

The Case of Aden Hailu

A second case, the case of Aden Hailu, arose in the spring of 2015. Hailu's was the first case to challenge whether the AAN guidelines adequately measure all functions of the entire brain, including the brain stem, under Nevada law.[39]

On April 1, 2015, Aden Hailu, a college student, went to Saint Mary's Regional Medical Center in Reno, Nevada, with abdominal pain.[40] During an exploratory laparotomy (a surgical procedure in which a large abdominal incision is made to allow direct observation of the abdominal organs), her appendix was removed, but she suffered "severe catastrophic anoxic, or lack of brain oxygen damage," and never woke up. Over two weeks she continued to have some brain function as documented by EEGs. On April 13 Dr. Heide, the director of neurology and stroke at Saint Mary's, examined Hailu and noted she was not brain dead but rapidly declining. On April 14 he stated that she no longer exhibited "indicia of neurological functioning." No repeat EEG was performed. An apnea test was performed six weeks later, on May 28, 2015, that confirmed "brain death unequivocally." On June 2 Saint Mary's told Hailu's father and guardian, Fanuel Gebreyes, that it intended to discontinue Hailu's ventilator. The court case made clear that the ventilator was to be discontinued because hospital personnel believed Hailu was dead based on brain criteria.

Gebreyes sought help from the courts to prevent the death pronouncement based on brain function loss. On June 18 the district court ruled that Gebreyes had until July 2, 2015, at 5:00 p.m. to have an independent neurologist examine Hailu. The district court ruled in Saint Mary's favor in July but delayed authorizing the discontinuation of the ventilator pending an appeal to the supreme court.

The Nevada Supreme Court refused to accept the lower court's finding that Hailu was dead. It noted that Nevada had adopted the UDDA in 1985. While the district court had determined that Saint Mary's physicians were justified in concluding Hailu was dead according to the AAN guidelines, the supreme court questioned whether the AAN guidelines were acceptable under the Nevada law defining death according to the UDDA.

The court raised two concerns. First, as we have noted, there are several potential criteria sets for measuring the death of the brain.

The AAN guidelines are a more recent set, but there are others tracing all the way back to the Harvard criteria. The Nevada law requires that the standards adopted be considered accepted medical standards by states that have adopted the UDDA.

The court held, "We are not convinced that the AAN guidelines have replaced the Harvard criteria as the accepted medical standard for states like Nevada that have enacted the UDDA." Here the hospital's failure to repeat the EEG becomes critical. The court seems to contend that the Harvard criteria require a flat EEG as a confirmatory test after the initial three tests (unresponsivity, absence of spontaneous movements and breathing, and absence of reflexes). There is good reason to believe that the Harvard criteria did not actually require the EEG. The additional test was suggested as a confirmation, but many commentators about the Harvard criteria, including Henry Beecher, the lead author, subsequently made the point that death can be pronounced on the basis of the initial three criteria without a confirmatory EEG. Furthermore, the AAN criteria clearly do not require a confirmatory EEG. Thus, when the hospital failed to repeat the EEG, it opened the door to the court's questioning about whether the use of the AAN criteria (without an EEG) meets the law's requirement that the standards for declaring death be the same as the standards used in other states that have adopted the UDDA. While the court claimed that it "does not attempt to replace its judgement for that of medical experts, nor does it attempt to set in stone certain medical criteria for determining brain death," it did state that Saint Mary's would need to establish that the AAN criteria set is accepted in other states. At this point it appeared that the hospital could provide such evidence when the case was heard again in the lower court.

The supreme court, however, raised a second issue, which would have been more difficult for the hospital. It pointed out that regardless of whether the AAN criteria are accepted in other states, the Nevada law requires that the tests must demonstrate the irreversible loss of all functions of the entire brain, including the brain stem. According to the supreme court, the literature shows that certain brain functions—hypothalamic secretions, posterior pituitary secretion of antidiuretic hormone, and thermoregulation—seem to remain after the standard tests for brain death have been met. The court said the hospital must provide expert testimony to demonstrate that the AAN guidelines establish "an irreversible cessation of . . . all functions of the person's entire brain, including his or her brainstem." The case was remanded back to the lower courts with an injunction to continue ventilator support. This case, then, directly challenged what criteria physicians use to determine irreversible cessation of all brain function. The case, however, became moot on January 5, 2016, when Hailu had a cardiac arrest and her heart could not be revived.[41]

Alternatives to the Whole-Brain Definition

The simple equation of brain death with "irreversible coma" by the Harvard committee should give us pause. Was it really the integrating capacity of the entire brain the committee members had in mind? If so, why did they substitute the term "irreversible coma"? There is another way to put the problem with a whole-brain definition of death. Can it really be true that some mere brain-stem reflex—the gag reflex, for example—can make the difference between being alive and being dead? The current whole-brain law implies that if one minor function survives, then the individual is alive, but without it, the individual is deceased. Can this view, taken literally, be defensible?

Several alternatives have been proposed to the whole-brain view. Depending on how we understand "integrating capacity," three other positions deserve special consideration. These are referred to as brain-stem death, somatic death, and higher-brain death. The latter two are the subjects of the next two chapters, but first, a word about so-called brain-stem death.

The British discussion of the definition of death focuses on "brainstem death" rather than the death of the whole brain. It is difficult to establish how important this distinction is. The attention given to the brain stem can be attributed largely to two influential British contributors to the discussion, Bryan Jennett and, especially, Christopher Pallis.[42] As Pallis puts it, "I conceive of human death as a state in which there is irreversible loss of the capacity for consciousness combined with irreversible loss of the capacity to breathe (and hence to maintain a heartbeat). Alone, neither would be sufficient. Both are essentially brain-stem functions (predominantly represented, incidentally, at different ends of the brain stem)."[43] Thus, although Pallis concludes that "the necessary and sufficient component of brain death is death of the brain stem,"[44] he focuses only on consciousness and respiration. In contrast, in May 2012 an international consortium was convened by Health Canada and Canadian Blood Services in collaboration with the World Health Organization to develop international guidelines for the determination of death. In a manuscript published in 2014, the group defined death to be "the permanent loss of capacity for consciousness and all brainstem functions."[45] Thus, both Pallis and this international consortium are focused on brain-stem functions, differing with respect to which brain-stem functions must be "irreversibly lost." Conversely, most American commentators have resisted the brain-stem formulation, insisting that all functions of the entire brain (including the brain stem) must be destroyed for death to occur. For example, the US President's Council on Bioethics in 2008 specifically said that brain-stem criteria are not sufficient for the declaration of brain death because, although a dead brain stem will nearly always indicate a dead higher brain, this would not be so in the case of a primary lesion of the brain stem.[46]

If the brain stem is destroyed, arousal may not be possible, but it seems plausible that the information of consciousness may still be stored in the higher-brain centers. It is at least theoretically possible that some functions related to mentation—dreaming, for example—may remain. Those who insist that death should be pronounced only if all brain functions are lost have been reluctant to accept death pronouncements based solely on brain-stem destruction.

Two problems with the Pallis notion of brain-stem death arise. First, as we have noted, it is theoretically possible that brain tissue above the brain stem, particularly the cerebrum, may still be alive and retain information considered important. This is also problematic for the 2012 international consortium. Second, defenders of brain-stem death, like Pallis, who are concerned only about consciousness and respiration have no reason to test for other brain-stem functions, such as the many reflexes mediated through this portion of the brain. Although the presence of the gag reflex or the eye blink reflex was sufficient for a defender of the Harvard criteria, advocates of the UDDA, and the international consortium working with the World Health Organization to consider someone alive, Pallis would not find such brain-stem-mediated nerve circuits intrinsically important.

In spite of clinical and conceptual differences between the whole-brain and brain-stem formulations, there is considerable agreement that the practical differences are minimal. The Americans, the British, and the new international consortium support the pronouncement of death based on the irreversible loss of neurological functions but consider someone alive who retains brain activity, including activity regulating respiration. The other two alternatives to the whole-brain concept of death—the somatic and higher-brain concepts of death—differ substantially. They are the subjects of the next two chapters.

Notes

1. Harvard Medical School, "A definition of irreversible coma: report of the Ad Hoc Committee of the Harvard Medical School to Examine the Definition of Brain Death," *JAMA* 1968;205(6):337–340.

2. Jonas H, "Philosophical reflections on human experimentation," *Daedalus* 1969;98(2):219–247.

3. Institute of Society, Ethics and the Life Sciences, Task Force on Death and Dying, "Refinements in criteria for the determination of death," *JAMA* 1972;221(1):48–53.

4. President's Commission for the Study of Ethical Problems in Medicine and Biomedical and Behavioral Research, *Defining Death: Medical, Legal and Ethical Issues in the Definition of Death* (Washington, DC: US Government Printing Office, 1981), 32–35.

5. Ibid., 33.

6. Bernat JL, Culver CM, Gert B, "On the definition and criterion of death," *Annals of Internal Medicine* 1981;94(3):389–394.

7. President's Commission, *Defining Death*, 2.

8. "Report of the medical consultants on the diagnosis of death to the President's Commission for the Study of Ethical Problems in Medicine and Biomedical and Behavioral Research," in President's Commission for the Study of Ethical Problems in Medicine and Biomedical and Behavioral Research, *Defining Death*, 157; Flowers WM, Patel BR, "Persistence of cerebral blood flow after brain death," *Southern Medical Journal* 2000;93(4):364–370.

9. Harvard Medical School, "Definition of irreversible coma," 337–338.

10. Mohandas A, Chou SN, "Brain death: a clinical and pathological study," *Journal of Neurosurgery* 1971;35(2):211–218.

11. In 1971 Beecher also excluded spinal reflexes. See Beecher HK, "The new definition of death. Some opposing views," *Internationale Zeitschrift für klinische Pharmakologie, Therapie, und Toxikologie* [International journal of clinical pharmacology, therapy, and toxicology] 1971;5(2):120–124.

12. "An appraisal of the criteria of cerebral death: a summary statement. A collaborative study," *JAMA* 1977;237(10):982–986.

13. Cranford RE, "Minnesota Medical Association criteria: brain death—concept and criteria, part I," *Minnesota Medicine* 1978;61(9): 561–563.

14. "Report of the medical consultants," 159–166.

15. American Academy of Pediatrics Task Force on Brain Death in Children, "Report of special task force. Guidelines for the determination of brain death in children," *Pediatrics* 1987;80(2):298–300.

16. Quality Standards Subcommittee of the American Academy of Neurology, "Practice parameters for determining brain death in adults: summary statement," *Neurology* 1995;45(5):1012–1014.

17. The President's Commission does, however, list severe illnesses and metabolic abnormalities (e.g., hepatic encephalopathy, hyperosmolar coma, and preterminal uremia) as confounding conditions to be excluded.

18. Academy of Medical Royal Colleges, *A Code of Practice for the Diagnosis and Confirmation of Brain Death* (London: Academy of Medical Royal Colleges, 2008).

19. Wijdicks EFM, Varelas PN, Gronseth GS, Greer DM; American Academy of Neurology, "Evidence-based guideline update: determining

brain death in adults: report of the Quality Standards Subcommittee of the American Academy of Neurology," *Neurology* 2010;74(23):1911–1918.

20. Nakagawa T, Ashwal S, Mathur M, Mysore M; Committee for Determination of Brain Death in Infants and Children, "Guidelines for the determination of brain death in infants and children: an update of the 1987 task force recommendations—executive summary," *Annals of Neurology* 2012;71(4):573–585.

21. Beecher, "New definition of death."

22. On pediatrics, see Mejia RE, Pollack MM, "Variability in brain death determination practices in children," *JAMA* 1995;274(7):550–553; Mathur M, Petersen L, Stadtler M, et al., "Variability in pediatric brain death determination and documentation in southern California," *Pediatrics* 2008;121(5):988–993; on adults, see Greer DM, Varelas PN, Haque S, Wijdicks E, "Variability of brain death determination guidelines in leading US neurologic institutions," *Neurology* 2008;70(4):284–289; Greer DM, Wang HH, Robinson JD, Varelas PN, Henderson GV, Wijdicks EF, "Variability of brain death policies in the United States," *JAMA Neurology* 2016;73(2):213–218.

23. "Appraisal of the criteria," 984.

24. Winkfield v. Children's Hospital Oakland, Case No. C13-5993, US District Court, Northern District of California Oakland, filed December 30, 2013, http://thaddeuspope.com/images/Mcmath_ND_Cal_12-30-13_.pdf.

25. Winkfield v. Rosen, First Amended Complaint for Damages for Medical Malpractice, Case No. Rg 15760730, Superior Court of the State of California for the County of Alameda, filed November 4, 2015. At the time of this writing, this court action has not been resolved. On January 8, 2016, both Children's Hospital of Oakland and Dr. Frederick Rosen filed for a demurrer; both were overruled on March 14, 2016, setting the stage for a court hearing in which Winkfield will have the opportunity to prove her child is now alive. See Spears v. Rosen, Demurrer and Motion to Strike Complaint Denied Superior Court of California, County of Alameda, Case No. RG15760730, filed March 14, 2016.

26. Winkfield v. Children's Hospital Oakland.

27. Matter of Jahi McMath, Superior Court of California, County of Alameda, No. RP13707598.

28. Winkfield v. Children's Hospital Oakland, Case No. C13-5993 SBA, US District Court for the Northern District of California, January 6, 2014.

29. DeBolt D, Bender KJ, Hurd R, "Jahi McMath: brain-dead teen's family moves her from Children's Hospital Oakland," *San Jose Mercury News*, January 5, 2014, www.mercurynews.com/breaking-news/ci _24852227/jahi-mcmath-leaves-childrens-hospital-oakland.

30. Shewmon DA, "Chronic 'brain death': meta-analysis and conceptual consequences," *Neurology* 1998;51(6):1538–1545.

31. Winkfield v. Rosen.

32. Wijdicks EF, *Brain Death* (Philadelphia PA: Lippincott, Williams and Wilkins, 2000), 29–43.

33. Schrader H, Krogness K, Aakvaag A, Sortland O, Purvis K, "Changes of pituitary hormones in brain death," *Acta Neurochirurgica* 1980;52(3–4):239–248; Goldie WD, Chiappa KH, Young RR, Brooks EB, "Brainstem auditory and short-latency somatosensory evoked responses in brain death," *Neurology* 1981;31(3):248–256.

34. Bernat JL, "Refinements in the definition and criterion of death," in *The Definition of Death: Contemporary Controversies*, ed. Youngner SJ, Arnold RM, Schapiro R (Baltimore, MD: Johns Hopkins University Press, 1999), 83–92.

35. See, for example, Halevy A, Brody B, "Brain death: reconciling definitions, criteria, and tests," *Annals of Internal Medicine* 1993;119(6): 519–525; Nair-Collins M, "Death, brain death, and the limits of science: why the whole-brain concept of death is a flawed public policy," *Journal of Law, Medicine & Ethics* 2010;38(3):667–683.

36. Shappell CN, Frank JI, Husari K, Sanchez M, Goldenberg F, Ardelt A, "Practice variability in brain death determination: a call to action," *Neurology* 2013;81(23):2009–2014; Citerio G, Murphy PG, "Brain death: the European perspective," *Seminars in Neurology* 2015;35(2):139–144; Greer et al., "Variability of brain death."

37. President's Commission, *Defining Death*, 2.

38. Burkle CM, Schipper AM, Wijdicks EF, "Brain death and the courts," *Neurology* 2011;76(9):837.

39. NRS 451.007 (Nevada Revised Statutes, Chapter 451, "Determination of Death").

40. In the Matter of the Guardianship of the person and estate of Aden Hailu, an adult, Fanuel Gebreyes, appellant, v. Prime Healthcare Services LLC, D/B/A St. Mary's Regional Medical Center, Supreme Court of the State of Nevada, No. 68531, 131 Nev Advance Opinion 89, filed November 16, 2015.

41. Sonner S, Ritter K, "Woman in Reno hospital end-of-life case dies on life support," *Providence Journal*, January 5, 2016.

42. Jennett B, "The donor doctor's dilemma: observations on the recognition and management of brain death," *Journal of Medical Ethics* 1975;1(2):63–66; Pallis C, "ABC of brain stem death: reappraising death," *British Medical Journal* 1982;285(6352):1409–1412; Pallis C, "ABC of brain stem death: from brain death to brain stem death," *British Medical Journal* 1982;285(6353):1487–1490; Pallis C, "ABC of brain stem death: the argument about the EEG, *British Medical Journal* 1983;286(6361):284–287.

43. Pallis, "ABC of brain stem death: reappraising," 1410.

44. Ibid., 1409. Almost identical views have been expressed by the Academy of Medical Royal Colleges in 1998 and 2008. See Academy of Medical Royal Colleges, *A Code of Practice for the Diagnosis of Brain Stem Death* (London: UK Department of Health, 1998); Academy of Medical Royal Colleges, *Code of Practice* (2008).

45. Shemie SD, Hornby L, Baker A, et al.; International Guidelines for Determination of Death Phase 1 Participants, "International guideline development for the determination of death," *Intensive Care Medicine* 2014;40(6):788–797.

46. US President's Council on Bioethics, *Controversies in the Determination of Death: A White Paper by the President's Council on Bioethics* (Washington, DC: US President's Council on Bioethics, 2008), 32.

4

The Circulatory, or Somatic, Concept of Death

One of the two major sets of alternatives to the whole-brain definition of death is a more traditional definition holding that death is somehow related to the irreversible loss of the flowing of essential bodily fluids—blood and breath. The standard American legal definition of death, based on the UDDA, includes two ways in which death can be determined: the direct measurement of the loss of all functions of the entire brain or the irreversible loss of circulatory and respiratory function.[1] That death can be determined based on the loss of circulatory and respiratory function has caused great confusion and has recently been the subject of increased attention.

A persistent minority of Americans and others has continued to insist that death is only properly understood as the irreversible loss of circulatory and respiratory function. Some come to this conclusion because of religious belief. Orthodox Jews, for example, relate life to breath and often deny that someone who has irreversibly lost brain function is dead if respiratory and circulatory functions remain. A number of sophisticated philosophers and physicians have also continued to hold this view.[2] Although precise numbers are difficult to determine, it seems likely that about 10 percent of the US population insists on some version of a circulatory definition of death.[3]

In the last chapter we described the case of Jahi McMath, a twelve-year-old girl who suffered severe bleeding after surgery for sleep apnea that led to a lack of oxygen flow to her brain at an Oakland hospital. Two different claims were made by Jahi's mother, Nailah Winkfield, and the attorney representing her. First, as we described in chapter 3, Winkfield disagreed that brain function was lost. This claim was repeated in an amended complaint filed in November 2015 before the Superior Court of the State of California for the County of Alameda.[4] Winkfield, however, also took the position that even if brain function had been lost, Jahi was not dead as long as circulation and respiration remained (even if the respiration was the result of ventilatory support).[5] Although Winkfield's position was a minority one, it should be apparent that there is no scientific basis for refuting it. Jahi's mother simply believes that her daughter should be treated as alive as long as she continues to respire and circulate blood.

Two Measurements of Death

This second basis for determining death—by measuring circulatory and respiratory function loss—introduces considerable ambiguity. It sounds like the traditional concept of death, which has variously been referred to as "cardiac," "circulatory," or "respiratory." At its worst, the inclusion in the law of both neurological and respirocirculatory means of pronouncing death has sometimes been understood as offering two different meanings of death, with the puzzling possibility that one could be simultaneously dead and alive—dead by one meaning, and alive by the other. For example, someone like Jahi McMath, with irreversible loss of all functions of the brain but with circulation and respiration retained mechanically, could be dead by brain criteria but alive by circulatory criteria.

Circulation as an Indicator of Brain-Based Death

More careful commentators have held that there can be only one meaning of death for the human being, although there could be two different methods of determining that death has occurred. The proponents of this single-meaning interpretation who accept some version of the brain-based concept of death, such as that in the UDDA, have generally held that humans should be deemed dead when all brain functions are irreversibly lost, but that there are two alternative ways of measuring that state. They claim that typically, it is sufficient to establish loss of circulatory and respiratory function. They note it is a biological fact that in the normal case, absence of circulation and respiration inevitably means the brain has been destroyed.

We need to be aware, however, that in special circumstances, it is possible that brain function has not been destroyed when circulation has been lost irreversibly. In the first seconds, perhaps minutes, after circulation has been lost, some brain functions may still be possible. Thus, though circulation loss is usually an indirect indicator of brain status, there may be exceptional circumstances when it is not.

If people look at circulation and respiration to determine whether brain function has been lost, they are merely using these measurements as a shortcut to establish the death of the brain tissue. Some, such as Alex Capron, claim that the meaning of "death" has always been the loss of bodily integrating capacity under the central control of the brain and that establishing irreversible loss of circulation and respiration has simply been a traditional and simple way of documenting the loss of that integrating capacity.[6]

Circulation Loss as Intrinsically Important

Others doubt that death has been understood throughout history as the loss of bodily integrating capacity. They hold that traditionally, human death has meant something like the irreversible loss of circulation and respiration—fluid flow. Apparently, Jahi McMath's mother holds this view—that circulation and respiration are intrinsically important—as she continues to claim her daughter is alive even though she at times acknowledges that brain function has been irreversibly lost.

The Meaning of Death Changed in the Late Twentieth Century

Among those who think that the loss of circulation and respiration is the traditional understanding of the concept of death, two views about what death has come to mean are possible. Some hold that in the late twentieth century, most people switched to a bodily integrating, neurological view of death. They still might rely on fluid flow loss as an indicator that someone has died, but not because circulation and respiration are intrinsically important. Rather, they would now look to fluid flow, much as Capron and others would, as a sign of loss of integrating capacity. If fluid flow has been lost in such a way that brain integrating capacity is destroyed (that is, brain tissues have ceased to function), then the loss of capacity to breathe and circulate blood is an indirect sign that death (that is, loss of brain function) has occurred.

Those who hold that loss of neurological integrating capacity has always been what we meant by death, and also those who hold that this has recently become the dominant view, would logically think that the loss of circulation is a measure of death (i.e., irreversible loss of brain-mediated bodily integrating capacity) only when circulation has been lost long enough for brain tissue to be destroyed. A few seconds of absence of cardiac activity would not count as death, because brain-based integrating capacity would not have been lost irreversibly. The critical empirical question for someone using cardiac arrest as an indirect measure of brain status would be, How long can the brain go without blood flow and still recover at least some of its integrating functions? In some cases a person has lost circulation for two to three minutes and had some level of brain function once circulation was restored. To be sure, such trauma to the brain might leave the individual with irreversible damage—perhaps to the level of an irreversible coma or PVS—but not with the complete loss of brain integrating capacity. For someone who looks at circulation loss as an indicator of irreversible loss of all brain function, the critical question is, How long a period of documented circulation loss is compatible with restoration of some integrative brain function? The answer is apparently at least several minutes.

The Meaning of Death Remains the Irreversible Loss of Fluid Flow

Still others (like Jahi McMath's mother), however, have clung to something like the fluid flow concept as intrinsically important to classifying humans as alive. They have held that people are alive as long as the capacity for fluid flow remains (even if it can be established that brain function is irreversibly lost). We can refer to this as the circulatory, or somatic, concept of death—the view that the presence of circulation is intrinsically important, regardless of brain status (we shall see why it is sometimes called somatic). Although data are difficult to come by, perhaps about 10 percent of Americans have stubbornly remained committed to this circulatory concept of death.[7] They believe that someone with circulating blood is alive, even if respiration is maintained by a ventilator or other means of artificial respiration. The individual is alive even if there is clear evidence of the irreversible loss of all brain function. For one who holds this view, a different empirical question is critical: How long can an individual endure loss of circulation and still have that circulation restored (even if brain function is not reestablished and therefore the brain's integrative activity is gone forever)?

In cases of potential organ procurement following death based on circulatory criteria, somewhat different questions are at stake for those who see circulation as an indirect indicator of brain function and those who see it as intrinsically important. Protocols for the donation of organs following circulatory death (typically abbreviated DCD, donation after circulatory death) require that death be established before organ procurement. Typically, these protocols involve a death pronouncement after a period of cardiac arrest long enough that circulation cannot be reestablished. As we have seen, it is critical whether this irreversibility is physiologically impossible or whether it is merely legally and morally impossible (because someone has refused attempts at resuscitation or life support).

DCD and Evidence of Death

The DCD protocols typically rely on mere legal irreversibility (sometimes now called permanent loss of function). The two different understandings of the role of circulation in establishing that death has occurred turn out to require two different criteria for establishing permanent loss, and therefore death.

Time until Brain Function Is Lost

For those who view circulation loss as only indirect evidence of the loss of brain function, the critical question, as we have seen, is, How long must circulation be lost to cause the irreversible loss of brain function? It turns out that very little attention has been devoted to this question. Clearly, the brain can go for a few minutes without circulation and still have at least some functions survive. Exactly how long is an empirical question that needs more attention. Anyone using loss of circulation as indirect evidence of the loss of brain function should be interested in this question.

Time until the Heart Cannot Restart Itself (Autoresuscitate)

For those who view circulation loss as intrinsically important, the critical question is, How long must circulation be lost before it cannot (or will not) be reestablished? In the context of a decision not to attempt resuscitation, this view that circulation is intrinsically important implies that circulation loss must be long enough so that autoresuscitation is not possible—that is, long enough so that the heart function will not restart spontaneously.

There is extensive literature trying to answer this question. The early DCD protocol at the University of Pittsburgh said after a 120-second period of asystole, one could conclude that a heart would not autoresuscitate.[8] The more conservative Institute of Medicine Committee on Organ Procurement and Transplant Policy suggested a period of five minutes.[9] Others, even more conservative, have insisted on as long as ten minutes.[10] These would be the times that one would have to wait before declaring death on the basis of circulatory criteria, assuming that the basis for pronouncing death was the intrinsic importance of circulation and the legal impossibility of a reversal occurring in the face of a valid refusal of attempts at resuscitation and life support. Logically, the possibility of autoresuscitation is important only if circulation per se is intrinsically important, not if we are using circulation as indirect evidence of brain status. It is quite possible that brain tissue could be destroyed from anoxia before (or after) autoresuscitation became impossible.

Circulatory Death and Organ Procurement

The concept of death based on circulatory criteria is important not only for those who believe that some people with dead brains may not be dead people but also for those who are interested in procuring organs from people who do not meet the tests for the irreversible loss of brain function. Because the criteria sets for establishing the loss of brain function generally require the repeating of tests over periods of six to twenty-four hours, many people who are pronounced dead by relying on traditional circulatory criteria do not qualify to be organ donors because of brain function loss. That has led many to consider procuring organs from those pronounced dead on the basis of circulatory criteria.

Two Kinds of Cases

Two groups of patients are considered feasible sources of organs following irreversible loss of circulation. The first group includes heart attack and accident victims who are brought to hospitals for emergency treatment. They suffer cardiac arrest before or after their arrival, and the attempted resuscitations fail. These people are eventually pronounced dead because of irreversible loss of circulatory function. These cases have come to be referred to as "unplanned" cases—that is, cases in which the stoppage of circulation was not planned.

The second group involves patients under care for critical illnesses who decide to exercise their right to refuse further life support. When that support is withdrawn, they will die. Because death is the expected outcome, these cases have been referred to as "planned" circulatory deaths. Some patients offer to become organ donors before the withdrawal of treatment. It is clearly illegal to take organs from dying individuals before they are declared dead; no organ procurement organization in the United States would do so. However, first the University of Pittsburgh Medical Center and now many other medical centers have developed protocols whereby such volunteer donors could be taken to the operating room before the withdrawal of life support so that as soon as the heart stops and death is pronounced, organs can be procured. Although the unplanned and planned groups raise somewhat different moral and policy issues, they are often considered together, as they are here.

It is striking that the death of the brain has become so ingrained as the "real" definition of death for organ procurement purposes that some, especially in Germany, have come to doubt that people who suffer irreversible cardiac arrest are really dead. In this vein, "only donation after brain death has been permitted by German law since 1997."[11] Nevertheless, American law states that death can be based on irreversible cessation of either circulatory or brain function.

Issues in Procuring Organs from Patients Considered Dead by Circulatory Criteria

In spite of the doubters, the majority of those who approve of any allograft organ transplantation agree that once proper permissions have been obtained, there is nothing ethically controversial about procuring organs from dead people, and that at least in the United States, it makes no difference in principle whether the death is measured by brain criteria or circulatory criteria. Individuals are just as dead either way. (Hence we plead that we not refer to individuals as "brain dead" or "heart dead." They should be thought of simply as "dead.")

The procurement of organs from asystolic patients who are dead—whether they are dead as a result of trauma, myocardial infarction, or a decision to forgo life support—appears at first not to present overwhelming problems. Nevertheless, some issues potentially add complexity to this apparently easily won consensus. Two of these are respecting the integrity of members of the procurement team and determining that the source of the organs is really dead.

The Rights and Welfare of the Caregivers

For reasons that are not entirely clear, some members of the health care team may be deeply troubled by procuring organs from recently deceased patients who are declared dead using circulatory criteria. They may be traumatized by the discontinuance of resuscitation efforts or termination of life support, the perfusion of the body, and the removal of organs from a still-warm body, in which, in some cases, a heart has beat only minutes previously. Some may have become so convinced that death should really be based on irreversible brain function loss that they are not satisfied that someone is dead when the death is measured using circulatory criteria.[12]

The emergency room and trauma team staff members will normally play only a preliminary role, assisting the patient and family in deciding to cease life support, participating in perfusion in the case of trauma and cardiac arrest patients, and preparing the body to be taken to the operating room in the case of patients with advance directives forgoing treatment. Even if there is a careful separation of the procurement team from other caregivers, the problems for professional staffs are potentially serious. Health care teams are normally militantly committed to attempting to prolong life, but they will be aware that in the case of unplanned arrests, others are standing by with very different objectives in mind, and that in the case of planned arrests, the purposeful cessation of treatment followed by organ procurement is being contemplated. Procurement team members will need to understand that they are dealing with a truly dead body. This will be particularly true in the moments preceding perfusion, when patients will feel warm and manifest some signs often taken to be signs of life.

Compassion for nurses and other professionals on the team requires careful preparation and ample opportunity for those who have reservations to withdraw from the perfusion and procurement processes. This may be particularly troublesome for emergency room staff members who may not be intimately involved with organ procurement on a daily basis. With care and compassion, these problems can probably be avoided.

The Organ Source Must Really Be Dead

A more difficult problem raised by procuring organs from those pronounced dead by circulatory criteria may turn out to be establishing exactly when these people are dead. Common wisdom used to suggest that though it was more difficult to measure death using brain criteria, measuring death using heart or circulation loss was straightforward. Now it appears that exactly the opposite may be the case.

The asystolic heart can surely be used as a measure of the death of the individual after prolonged asystole, but there are important reasons why death should be pronounced (and organs procured) as quickly as possible. The Pittsburgh protocol in its original form called for a death pronouncement after two minutes of asystole. At this point, the protocol claimed, autoresuscitation was impossible, but it cannot be denied that cardioversion still could be accomplished mechanically. As we have seen, it is debatable whether a heart's stoppage should be considered "irreversible" if it could be restarted but will not be because a decision has been made not to do so and, in fact, in the case of a valid treatment-refusing advance directive, it would actually be illegal to attempt resuscitation. This is what we have referred to as the difference between physiological and legal irreversibility, and what others have referred to as the difference between irreversible and permanent loss of function.

Even more perplexing is whether an individual should be considered dead during the period when a heart could be restarted by people with expert skills and sophisticated equipment if those people and equipment are not available. The concept of irreversibility has suddenly become much more complex. Moreover, depending on the exact meaning of irreversibility, the brain tissue is not necessarily dead at the point when the heart is determined to be stopped irreversibly. In Pittsburgh a patient could, after two minutes, be called dead while his brain continued to live; this problem is addressed later. If the concept of death actually refers to the state in which the body no longer functions as an integrated whole and if functioning as an integrated whole requires brain activity, then the exact moment of irreversible circulation loss is not precisely when integrated functioning of the body as a whole is lost.

The significance of these subtle distinctions is not necessarily great in cases where the patient or surrogate has made an advance decision not to resuscitate, but in patients suffering unexpected cardiac arrest, this could raise serious problems. The initial working presumption of the trauma team must be that resuscitation should be pursued. Longer periods of asystole would be necessary to establish irreversibility, and therefore, there may be longer periods of warm ischemic time. This means that ethically, there must be a sharp separation of responsibility between the organ procurement team and the resuscitation team. This could mean that a longer period of asystole will be necessary to establish that the heart has really ceased function irreversibly (and has done so long enough to cause irreversible brain function loss, if that is the understanding of what it means to be dead). If the resuscitation team has been trying unsuccessfully for a long time to resuscitate, the heart may be asystolic for much more than two minutes. Having organ procurement on the agenda creates an incentive to cut resuscitation time because more lengthy attempts could diminish the value of organs. Regardless, according to current law, if the heart is really dead (however "dead" is defined), the dead donor rule will be satisfied (or will be satisfied as soon as enough time has passed for brain destruction to occur). Because the organs can survive as much as thirty minutes of warm ischemia, shifting to a longer period of asystole—say, five minutes—probably need not pose an insurmountable problem.

A more serious question lurks beneath the surface, however. Although there is a clear recognition in statutory definitions of death that death may be pronounced on the basis of irreversible loss of either circulatory or brain activity, the possibility of organ procurement based on death pronouncement following short periods of asystole poses a new challenge. Especially if asystolic periods as brief as two minutes are used for pronouncing death (on the basis of the irreversible loss of circulatory function), it seems likely that the brain tissue is really not dead at this moment. In fact, much of the literature advocating such death pronouncements does not even present firm evidence that the patient is unconscious. The vision of pronouncing a patient dead after only two minutes of asystole (while brain tissue still lives) starkly poses the question of whether someone really ought to be considered dead if the brain tissue is still alive. The asystolic organ source may force the participants in the definition-of-death debate to reconsider whether someone can be pronounced dead on the basis of the loss of circulatory function alone.

It had previously been assumed that if irreversible cardiac arrest occurred, then all brain functions would necessarily have ceased. That turns out to be not quite true. If brains can function even briefly after irreversible circulatory arrest, then society must reassess whether it should continue to accept a policy according to which death can occur when either circulatory or brain function is lost. This challenges society to reexamine whether it wants to treat people as dead when brain function exists. Of course, in routine cases of prolonged circulatory arrest, we could continue to pronounce death without measuring brain function. Surely all brain function has been destroyed with prolonged circulation stoppage. But in planned arrest we may want to insist that enough time pass following circulatory arrest not only to foreclose the possibility of autoresuscitation but also to ensure the irreversible loss of brain function.

The reasonable conclusion seems to be that, quite to our surprise, the emergence of donation after circulatory death has challenged our established definition that states simply that death may be pronounced when there is irreversible loss of either brain or circulatory function. From the point of view of those who hold the now-mainstream view that death is the irreversible loss of all brain functions, this received position should be amended to make clear that if circulatory function loss is used as an indicator of death, it must be only because it is an accurate predictor that brain function has been irreversibly lost, not because the loss of circulatory function per se is significant. It is becoming more and more clear, at least to those who advocate brain-based death pronouncement, that it is the brain's function that is critical, not the beating heart. Thus, if we can interpret irreversibility to mean "will not start again" rather than "cannot be started again," we still must use irreversible circulatory function loss to pronounce death only when the loss accurately measures the irreversible loss of brain function. Two minutes of asystole does not do this. Some longer time does. The neurologists need to tell us exactly how long the heart function must be stopped in order to say safely that the brain will never function again. Five minutes of asystole appears to be a much safer period than two minutes. Perhaps even a longer time is necessary.

Conversely, for the minority who have persistently held, or have reverted to, the view that death means irreversible loss of bodily integrative functions independent of the brain—those who opt for Shewmon's view (see the following) or the view of the minority of the US President's Council on Bioethics—then it really is irreversibility of circulation that is critical, whatever the state of the brain at that point.

The DCD Protocols

Three developments involving DCD protocols implicitly rely on different interpretations of what it means to be dead by circulatory or cardiac criteria. Let us briefly consider each development.

The Infant Heart Transplant Cases

A controversial protocol at the University of Colorado was designed to procure hearts for transplant from newborn infants with conditions incompatible with life. Often referred to as the Boucek protocol (after the head of the team that developed it), it identified infants whose parents had made independent, valid decisions to forgo life support.[13] The investigators withdrew life support, waited for circulatory arrest, and then waited further for a period chosen to establish the impossibility of autoresuscitation. For the first case, they waited three minutes; for the second and third cases, they waited only seventy-five seconds. Death was pronounced, the hearts were procured, and then they were transplanted. The investigators found that the hearts could be restarted and function successfully.

Several problems arose that are relevant to the concept of death. First, it should be clear that waiting enough time to rule out autoresuscitation is plausible only if the legal and moral impossibility of restoration of circulation is intrinsically important. It does not establish that circulation could not be restored with intervention. (In fact, the restoration of heart function following transplant implies that it could be restored.)

There were more problems. No consensus, peer-reviewed criteria existed for establishing the waiting time to rule out autoresuscitation in newborns. Hence, even the three-minute wait time, which is arguably within the range of the standard of practice for adults, cannot be assumed for children.[14] Even if the three-minute time were defensible, moving to seventy-five seconds of asystole was without precedent.

Moreover, we have seen that many people would rely on evidence of a lack of circulation as indirect evidence that the brain has irreversibly lost its capacity to function. Even if the three-minute or seventy-five-second waiting time was somehow found to be sufficient to rule out autoresuscitation, it surely is not sufficient time to presume that brain function was lost. If one is relying on the irreversible loss of circulation as indirect evidence of brain function loss, this would certainly be an error in this case. Surely, brain function was not irreversibly lost in seventy-five seconds, and plausibly, the capacity for brain function was not lost in three minutes.

These cases also raise the question of what precisely is meant by cessation of circulatory function. The investigators made clear that the heart function was restored (albeit in another infant who received the transplant). Some of us raised the question of whether it can be said that cardiac function ceased irreversibly if the plain evidence was that heart function was restored.[15]

The members of the Boucek team defended their action by claiming that the restoration of heart function was irrelevant because death was pronounced based on establishing the irreversible loss of circulatory function. The infants pronounced dead never had their circulation restored and therefore were dead by circulatory criteria. Even if we assume that irreversibility is based on the legal impossibility of restarting circulation in infants with a valid decision to withdraw life support, it is clear that a more precise articulation is required of what it means for circulation to cease. The authors of the early legal definitions of death, such as the UDDA, never faced the question of whether loss of circulation followed by restoration of heart function so that it maintains circulation in another body would still count as irreversible loss of circulation.

This raises a complex question: Did Boucek and colleagues believe that autoresuscitation would be impossible after either 180 or 75 seconds when they chose those time intervals to wait after asystole before pronouncing death? This belief, if empirically supported, would be grounds for claiming death, provided that circulation were independent not only of the restoration of heart function but also of the question of whether brain tissue were still alive. Conversely, if irreversible circulation loss is merely a basis for determining the status of the brain, there is no reason to assume that the infants pronounced dead after 180 or 75 seconds of asystole had irreversibly lost all brain functions. Quite to the contrary, there is strong reason to believe that the brain tissue is not dead and in fact retains the capacity to perform certain functions after 75 seconds and possibly after even 180 seconds. This is especially true for infants, whose brains are more resilient than those of adults. Pronouncing death in the Boucek cases requires the controversial assumption that death can be pronounced when circulation has irreversibly ceased (not counting the heart circulating blood in another body), regardless of the fact that the infants' brains undoubtedly retain a capacity to perform at least some functions. If death by circulatory criteria is based merely on the claim that circulation loss is indirect evidence of brain status, the Boucek infants could not be considered deceased at the time death was pronounced. The protocol requires that circulation loss is intrinsically the determiner of death, that the continued function of the heart to provide circulation outside the body can be ignored, that as little as seventy-five seconds of asystole is sufficient to claim the impossibility of autoresuscitation (without a peer-reviewed consensus), and that this interval can be used for newborns in addition to adults.

The New York City DCD Protocol

Although Boucek and his colleagues were making claims implying that they viewed circulation as intrinsically the sign of life (and its loss, death), another protocol designed to obtain organs from heart attack victims who were the subjects of unsuccessful rescue attempts by emergency responders took a different approach. Those behind this protocol seemed to defend their work by assuming that circulation did not matter as long as heart function had ceased. A report from the New York City UDCDD (Unplanned Donation after Circulatory Determination of Death) Study Group seems to rely on assumptions that contradict the Boucek group.

The NYC UDCDD group was attempting to develop a social consensus about pronouncing the death of heart attack victims for whom resuscitation was unsuccessful.[16] After the failed resuscitation and death pronouncement based on cardiocirculatory arrest by the rescue squad, a second team would be standing by; this second team would intervene to provide maximal effort to preserve organs (other than the heart) so that transport to a hospital could take place in such a way that the organs could be procured. To maximize organ preservation, the second team would offer cardiac massage and extracorporeal membrane oxygenation (ECMO). This would, in effect, restore circulation, which raises the question of whether the heart attack victim had actually experienced irreversible loss of circulation. Their defense was that as long as the heartbeat was not restored, the reestablishment of circulation did not matter.

This seems to be an obvious contradiction to the reasoning of the Boucek team. Boucek's group said that reestablishing a heartbeat did not matter because circulation was critical; the New York group said that reestablishing circulation did not matter because the heart was critical. Now, for the first time, we need to know precisely what it is about the circulatory system that would permit us to pronounce death. Is it the irreversible loss of circulation (as Boucek's group claims) or the irreversible loss of a heartbeat (as the New York group claims)?

The Michigan ECMO Project

The story gets even more complicated, however. A group at the University of Michigan has experimented with ECMO for many important uses in medicine. This group applied ECMO technology to preserve organs for transplant.[17] Its members were aware, however, that a reestablishment of circulation would raise questions about whether patients were dead. To avoid reanimation, they devised an ingenious plan of inserting catheters in the carotid arteries with balloons that could be inflated so that the ECMO would restore circulation to the body but not to the head. Hence, the brain would be allowed to deteriorate without the supply of oxygen that would otherwise come from the ECMO. They defended their approach by claiming that because the restoration of circulation did not reanimate the brain, the recipients of the ECMO were still dead. Obviously, this defense works only if one views absence of circulation as evidence of brain status. The recipients of the ECMO would be dead if, and only if, circulation were indirect evidence of brain status, not if circulation to the body were intrinsically important.

Both those who believe that circulation is intrinsically important and those who believe that it is important as indirect evidence of the loss of the body's integrating capacity have referred to this basis for pronouncing death as "circulatory death." In the past decade a new understanding of death pronouncement based on circulation loss has emerged. It views circulation loss not as evidence of brain function loss but rather as the loss of the body's capacity to perform integrated functions independent of the brain. This position, articulated best by Alan Shewmon, deserves careful attention.

Shewmon's Somatic Concept

The most influential advocate for something resembling the circulatory concept of death is the neurologist Alan Shewmon. He has accepted the concept of death as the irreversible loss of bodily integrating capacity, but he notes that "most somatically integrative functions of the body are not brain-mediated."[18] He claims that substantial capacity for such integration continues to be possible, even in the absence of brain function. He points out that a body with a completely destroyed brain can be maintained (albeit with considerable medical support) and that with maintenance of ventilatory support and proper nutrition and hydration, many systemic, complex integrative functions remain possible. He cites homeostasis, elimination, energy balance, maintenance of body temperature, wound healing, fighting of infections, development of febrile response, cardiovascular and hormonal stress responses, successful gestation of a fetus, sexual maturation of a child, and proportional growth as capacities that have all been maintained in a so-called brain-dead body.[19] He has persuasively argued that if somatic integrating capacities are what are critical for determining whether a human body is dead or alive, then it is clear that the mere death of the brain cannot be taken as human death.

Thus, Shewmon has put forward a somatic concept of death that identifies a wide range of integrative body functions, not merely circulation and respiration. Nevertheless, he associates his position with the traditional respiratory and circulatory definition of death, noting that "both *circulation* and *respiration* (in the technical, biochemical sense linked to energy generation) are presupposed as means to many, if not all, of the above functions" (italics in the original).[20] Therefore, there is a close compatibility between his somatic concept of death and the views of those who adhere to the more traditional circulatory and respiratory definitions, at least those who hold that we have looked to circulation and respiration in pronouncing death because these functions have been considered intrinsically important (and not mere indirect indicators of brain status).

The result has been that over the past decade more doubt has arisen about the whole-brain-based definition of death than was anticipated in the last decades of the twentieth century. Now, not only those who traditionally thought circulation and respiration were an intrinsic sign of life but also those who adopt the more sophisticated somatic integrative concept—including some who would nevertheless accept procuring of life-prolonging organs from certain people before their deaths, that is, those who have come to reject the dead donor rule—are unwilling to accept the whole-brain basis for pronouncing the death of humans.[21] Those who hold this view still represent a small minority in the United States and most other Western countries. The view, however, has gained more credibility lately, as seen by the seriousness with which it was taken by the US President's Council on Bioethics.

The Two Definitions of the US President's Council on Bioethics

The US President's Council on Bioethics has identified two different definitions of death. One of these definitions—referred to as "position one"—rejects a neurologically based definition and closely follows Shewmon's work. Position one was adopted by two of the council's eighteen members (Alfonso Gomez-Lobo and council chair Edmund D. Pellegrino)—closely mirroring the estimated 10 percent of the US population that has never accepted neurological definitions.[22]

Having been challenged by Shewmon's persuasive claim that many bodily integrative functions exist outside the brain and that they remain possible even after the death of the brain, the majority of the President's Council has nevertheless adopted a brain-oriented definition of death, which is referred to as "position two." It has identified more or less the same group as dead as was singled out by the view that assumed the brain was responsible for bodily integrative functions but has offered a new conceptual foundation for this view. The majority have claimed that a more compelling view of a body functioning as a whole requires "the work of self-preservation, achieved through the organism's need-driven commerce with the surrounding world."[23] This interaction with the surrounding world requires the functioning of the brain, and thus the council's majority view provides a new basis for the defense of the neurological standard—what we have referred to as the whole-brain basis for pronouncing death.

This new level of complexity in defining death and differentiating the various roles that circulation might play in death pronouncement has created a much more complicated and confusing set of issues for death pronouncement in relation to organ procurement. This is particularly true for organ procurement that can be associated with death pronouncement based on circulatory or somatic death.

Although the circulatory or somatic view has gained some status in the past few years in its conflict with the whole-brain view, the more neurologically oriented definition of death that insists on the irreversible loss of all brain functions has also met competition from another, more liberal view: the higher-brain view. We now turn to this third major definition.

Notes

1. President's Commission for the Study of Ethical Problems in Medicine and Biomedical and Behavioral Research, *Defining Death: Medical, Legal and Ethical Issues in the Definition of Death* (Washington, DC: US Government Printing Office, 1981), 2.

2. Miller FG, Truog RD, *Death, Dying, and Organ Transplantation* (New York: Oxford University Press, 2012); Lamb D, *Death, Brain Death and Ethics* (Albany: State University of New York Press, 1985); Shewmon DA, "The brain and somatic integration: insights into the standard biological rationale for equating 'brain death' with death," *Journal of Medicine and Philosophy* 2001;26(5):457–478.

3. See Siminoff LA, Burant C, Youngner SJ, "Death and organ procurement: public beliefs and attitudes," *Kennedy Institute of Ethics Journal* 2004;14(3):217–234.

4. Winkfield v. Rosen, First Amended Complaint for Damages for Medical Malpractice, Case No. Rg 15760730, Superior Court of the State of California for the County of Alameda, filed November 4, 2015. At the time of this writing, this court action has not been resolved.

5. This case description is based on the work of Wells J, "Mother of brain-dead Jahi McMath defends ventilator decision," *Los Angeles Times*, February 24, 2014, http://articles.latimes.com/2014/feb/24/local/la -me-ln-mother-jahi-mcmath-defends-decision-20140224; Onishijan N, "A brain is dead, a heart beats on," *New York Times*, January 3, 2014, www.nytimes.com/2014/01/04/us/a-brain-is-dead-a-heart-beats-on .html?_r=1; Veatch RM, "Let parents decide if teen is dead," CNN, January 2, 2014, www.cnn.com/2014/01/02/opinion/veatch-defining -death/. See also Winkfield v. Rosen.

6. Capron AM, Kass LR, "A statutory definition of the standards for determining human death: an appraisal and a proposal," *University of Pennsylvania Law Review* 1972;121(2):114. See also President's Commission, *Defining Death*, 40–41. Capron was executive director of the commission.

7. Siminoff et al., "Death and organ procurement."

8. "University of Pittsburgh Medical Center Policy and Procedure Manual," *Kennedy Institute of Ethics Journal* 1993;3(2):A-1–A-15.

9. Institute of Medicine, Committee on Organ Procurement and Transplantation Policy, *Organ Procurement and Transplantation: Assessing Current Policies and the Potential Impact of the DHHS Final Rule* (Washington, DC: National Academy Press, 1999).

10. Koffman G, Gambaro G, "Renal transplantation from non-heart-beating donors: a review of the European experience," *Journal of Nephrology* 2003;16(3):334–341; Bos MA, "Ethical and legal issues in non-heart-beating organ donation," *Transplantation* 2005;79(9):1143–1147.

11. Fischer-Fröhlich CL, "Factors limiting organ donation in Baden-Württemberg," *Clinical Transplantation* 2013;27(Suppl 25):1.

12. Ibid.

13. Boucek MM, Mashburn C, Dunn SM, et al.; Denver Children's Pediatric Heart Transplant Team, "Pediatric heart transplantation after declaration of cardiocirculatory death," *New England Journal of Medicine* 2008;359(7):709–714.

14. Bernat J, "The boundaries of organ donation after circulatory death," *New England Journal of Medicine* 2007;359(7):669–671.

15. Veatch RM, "Donating hearts after cardiac death: reversing the irreversible," *New England Journal of Medicine* 2008;359(7):672–673.

16. Wall SP, Kaufman BJ, Gilbert AJ, et al.; NYC UDCDD Study Group, "Derivation of the uncontrolled donation after circulatory determination of death protocol for New York City," *Transplantation Proceedings* 2011;11(7):1417–1426.

17. Magliocca JF, Magee JC, Rowe SA, et al., "Extracorporeal support for organ donation after cardiac death effectively expands the donor pool," *Journal of Trauma: Injury, Infection, and Critical Care* 2005;58(6):1095–1102.

18. Shewmon, "Brain and somatic integration," 467.

19. Ibid., 467–468.

20. Ibid., 489.

21. See, e.g., Miller and Truog, *Death, Dying*.

22. US President's Council on Bioethics, *Controversies in the Determination of Death: A White Paper by the President's Council on Bioethics* (Washington, DC: US President's Council on Bioethics, 2008), 99 and 114.

23. Ibid., 60.

5

The Higher-Brain Concept of Death

The difficulties in developing a coherent whole-brain-based definition of death have raised problems not only for those who identify somatic integrative functions outside the brain but also for those who question whether literally all brain functions must be lost irreversibly before a neurologically based death pronouncement. Authors have noted that some brain functions may remain in patients who meet all the criteria in the standard sets of criteria for the death of the brain.[1] In particular, Halevy and Brody found that neurohormonal functioning, such as anterior pituitary hormone levels, has been observed as have delta, theta, and alpha EEG readings as well as brain-stem-evoked potentials.[2] Shewmon, in cataloging problems with whole-brain-based notions of death, not only points to integrative functions mediated outside the brain but also summarizes claims that have been made against the criteria sets used for brain-based death pronouncement.[3] Thus, there exist "functions" in some brains that supposedly meet the criteria for brains that have irreversibly lost all functions. This type of contradiction has reemerged in the case of Jahi McMath, whose family claims that evidence of hypothalamic hormonal secretions shows she is not dead by brain criteria.[4] There are two plausible responses to this paradox. The most straightforward would be to revise the criteria to make sure that hormonal and electrical functions are absent before death is pronounced. If the law requires all functions of the brain to be gone, then all functions ought to be tested. The alternative is to acknowledge that when the original proponents of brain-based death pronouncement put forward the standard that "all functions" must be lost, they really did not have in mind hormonal or electrical functions of the kind that Halevy, Brody, and others have identified. In fact, in the years since these paradoxical findings have become known, deaths based on brain function loss have continued to be pronounced using the same criteria sets that were in use before we were aware of this issue.

Ignoring these hormonal and electrical functions is not the only example of brain-death defenders excluding certain activities as too trivial to consider. James Bernat, the best-known defender of the whole-brain, bodily integrating–capacity definition of death, has acknowledged that we should include only the "critical" functions, excluding certain "nests of cells" as not sufficiently important.[5] Thus, he ends up defending the "whole-brain" concept while acknowledging that some functions can be ignored.

Similarly, Pallis, in defending the brain-stem concept, while suggesting that it is functionally equivalent to the whole-brain concept, identifies only consciousness and respiration as critical functions, permitting one to ignore all other brain functions, including not only the hormonal and electrical ones but also other brain-stem reflexes.[6]

If one is to retain a neurologically based concept of death, it is terribly implausible to insist that all brain functions must be lost irreversibly. Every reasonable defender of brain-based death pronouncement must exclude some functions, opening up the question of just which functions should be excluded.

Henry Beecher, the Harvard committee chairman, in a 1970 lecture defending brain-based death pronouncement (what we would call the "whole-brain" view), made clear which functions he deemed essential, and he did not seem to include all the brain's functions.[7] He believed that a human is dead when there is irreversible loss of the human's "personality, his conscious life, his uniqueness, his capacity for remembering, judging, reasoning, acting, enjoying, worrying, and so on." Beecher went on to argue, "We have proof that these and other functions reside in the brain. . . . It seems clear that when the brain no longer functions, when it is destroyed, so also is the individual destroyed; he no longer exists as a person; he is dead."[8] Certainly this conclusion follows from what we know about the brain, but there is a fundamental error in the argument. We have suggested that if there is a practical problem with the more conservative heart- and lung-oriented concepts, it is that they occasionally produce false positive tests for life. Some patients with circulatory function actually have irreversibly lost all brain functions. If the argument is to be made for brain-oriented criteria at all, then certainly this argument must be subject to the same criticism. The functions mentioned by Beecher and summarized by the term "irreversible coma" certainly are in the brain but clearly do not exhaust the brain's functions. Patients we would now say are in an irreversible coma, and also those who are in a PVS (what is also referred to as "unresponsive wakefulness syndrome"[9]), have purportedly irreversibly lost all the functions that Beecher enumerated but do not have dead brains. Focusing on the destruction of the whole brain may involve additional nonessential functions, just as focusing on the heart and lungs did. The hormonal and electrical activities identified by Halevy and Brody, along with any other insignificant nests of cells referred to by Bernat, would surely qualify.

Which Brain Functions Are Critical?

If every reasonable defender of a neurologically based concept of death needs to exclude some brain functions, the critical question is, which ones? Which brain functions are so important that their presence is a sign of life? Several candidates for functions critical to human existence have been proposed. Let us review them.

The Capacity for Rationality

Beecher's list of characteristics includes the human's ability to reason. The Latin name for our species, Homo sapiens, clearly implies that reasoning capacity is somehow an essential characteristic. Could it be that it is reasoning capacity, rather than integrating capacity, that is essential? Our considered moral judgments about those members of the species who do not have any capacity for reasoning but retain consciousness is that they are still to be considered living in a very real way. They are still to have human rights, protected by both moral and positive law.

Babies—lacking a language, a culture, and a capacity to reason—certainly are living in a human sense, even though they have never executed the reasoning function. One might, of course, argue that babies have the potential for reasoning—the capacity for future reasoning. In this sense they might be included among the category of living humans. But what about people afflicted with senile dementia, those with severe cognitive disabilities, or the apparently permanently psychotic? They also lack a capacity for rationality; in some cases they never have had that capacity, and in other cases they will never regain it. Yet it is clear that they are still living in a meaningful sense of the term. In fact, one of the great dangers of moving to any brain-oriented concept of death is that it might place us on a slippery slope leading to the eventual exclusion of certain individuals who lack a certain minimal quality of life from the category of the human. Unless this tendency can be avoided, the dangers of movement to brain-oriented concepts may well exceed the moral right-making tendencies. Whatever may be our propensity to see rationality as the pinnacle of human functioning, it must not be the characteristic that is essential to consider humans living. We must look elsewhere.

Personhood or Personal Identity

Some contributors to the definition-of-death discussion equate the loss of personhood or loss of personal identity with death.[10] Green and Wikler, for example, claim that continuity of personal identity is essential for the existence of a person. When continuity of personal identity ends, that person no longer exists.[11] This must surely be wrong as well. Assuming we are using the standard nonmoral definition of a person as a self-aware being, it is easy to recognize that there are human, living nonpersons—that is, humans who lack the capacity for self-awareness—who are nevertheless alive.[12] Even if continuity of personal identity ceases, a human—the same human—still exists. Infants, the severely senile, and perhaps other humans lack self-awareness yet surely are not dead. When advanced Alzheimer's disease patients have completely lost continuity of personal identity with their earlier existence, they continue to exist. It is not even plausible to say that they cease to be the people they once were. Everyone would recognize that patients who, through injury or illness, lose all continuity of personal identity—even those who could never regain that personal identity—are nevertheless the same individual. Their spouses would still be married to them, their health insurance would still cover their medical costs, they would still be the owners of their property, and so forth. Any other position would produce chaos. The "new individual" in the "old person's body" would own no assets, have no family, and have no insurance coverage. Such an individual is not only not dead; he or she is still the same individual (even if philosophers might say he or she is no longer a "person" in the sense of being self-aware or having continuity of personal identity).

The Capacity to Experience

Most of the other functions mentioned in lists of essentially human characteristics—consciousness and capacity for remembering, enjoying, worrying, acting voluntarily—characterize the human as an experiential animal. Experience is here taken in the broadest sense. Humans experience cognitively and emotionally. They cathect, comprehend, and experience through sense organs and through much more complex experiential modes. It seems clear that a human who has some vestige of consciousness, some capacity to experience in this broadest sense, could never be considered dead. To be sure, this human life may not be on the highest plane. It may be limited to a blurred vision of reality and stunted emotional experience, but it is nevertheless life of a form sufficiently human to be protected. Death behavior for such an individual is inappropriate.

Anencephalic infants are children born without functioning cerebral hemispheres, and therefore they never experience any consciousness. Although they are sometimes referred to as "brain absent," they may have a fully or partially functioning brain stem, such that they may have spontaneous respiration and therefore are living, unconscious beings by whole-brain standards. Still, they will never have the capacity to experience others or to have social interaction.[13]

The anencephalic infant and other humans without any capacity for consciousness raise the question of whether a being should be considered living if body functions such as respiration, circulation, digestion, and excretion are possible but consciousness is not. We saw in chapter 4 that the defenders of the somatic view answer in the affirmative, but most advocates for the higher-brain view would claim that without experience—consciousness—an essential element of the being is impossible. They hold that life—for purposes of public policy—requires this capacity to experience, or something very similar.

The Capacity for Social Interaction

Although humans may be experiential, they are also social creatures. At least in the Western tradition, the human's capacity to relate to fellow humans is a fundamental characteristic—some would even say essential. Is it meaningful to speak of a living human who lacks the capacity for social interaction? We must make clear that we are not at all saying that actual social interaction must take place for a creature to be alive. We are not even saying that such interaction must have ever taken place. To say this would place the human's existence at the mercy of fellow humans. The cruel treatment of a baby who has been abandoned in a room with no human interaction should not define that baby out of existence. Presumably the capacity for social interaction nevertheless remains.

Likewise, there are cases of feral children. People have occasionally found a child that has grown up in the forest with animals. These children are called feral children. If they have no social human interaction their whole childhood, they would act as animals do—they would bite, scratch, growl, and walk on all fours. They would not be able to talk or even know that any language existed. They would drink by lapping up water, eat grass, and eat raw meat. They would not know what was considered right or wrong and would not be able to conform to the norms of society. Similarly, children with severe autism have severely constrained capacity to experience others. It seems likely that even these extreme cases do not represent literally a complete lack of capacity for social interaction, no matter how stunted that capacity may be. Thus, we would insist on what is perhaps obvious: all of these children are living human beings. However, if there ever were a genetic human with literally no capacity to interact socially, the question of whether the individual would be considered a member of the human moral community arises.

What, then, is the relationship between the capacity for experience and the capacity for social interaction? It is conceivable that a condition could exist that would differentiate the two capacities. But to be able to experience but not interact with others would certainly be a bizarre form of existence. One of the most important experiences that humans have is social interaction. At least in the Western tradition, the human's capacity to relate to fellow humans is fundamental and integral to what we mean when we talk about what it means to be human. In fact, one could propose replacing the more traditional concepts of death (those focusing on the departure of the soul, or the irreversible cessation of fluid flow, or somatic integrating capacity), focusing instead on the irreversible loss of the capacity for experience or social interaction, rather than the irreversible loss of the body's integrating capacity. If this is the case, the implications for the whole-brain-oriented criteria for death are great.

What emerges is what is sometimes called a "higher-brain" concept of death, one that requires only the higher, or important, brain functions to be present for one to be considered alive. The term "higher" is, of course, ambiguous and vague. It suggests that only certain brain functions are more important. These may also be higher in anatomical location. Exactly what higher functions are critical and where those functions are located is a matter of philosophical and public policy decision.

Embodiment of Capacity

Is it simply capacity for experience and social interaction per se, or must there also be some embodiment of the capacity? Consider the bizarre and purely hypothetical case in which all of the information of the human brain is transferred to a computer hard drive, together with sufficient sensory inputs and outputs to permit some form of rudimentary experiential and social function. Would the deleting of the disk information be murder? This thought is so novel that perhaps we cannot even conceive clearly of the philosophical significance of the question. Certain worldviews influenced by the Greeks consider the mind the critical part of human existence. Liberation from the body—the flesh—is a goal. If all that is critical is mental, then presumably humans could, in theory, exist as computers.

Viewing the mind as the only essential feature of a human being, one of us has suggested, is the mistake of the "mentalists."[14] The mentalists accept that an individual could, in theory, exist completely disembodied. It seems quite possible, however, that our concept of the essential must include some embodiment. An adult male whose mind was transferred to a little girl's body would not be the continuing existence of the adult male; it would be a chimera, a combination of two beings—something we hope would never be created. The human is, after all, something more than a sophisticated computer. At least in the Judeo-Christian tradition, the body is an essential element, not something from which humans escape in liberation. If this is the case, then the essential element is embodied capacity for experience and social interaction. According to this view, if either the mind or the body ceases to exist (even if the mind were to continue to exist in another body, or even if the body continued to exist without a mind), that individual would no longer exist. He or she would be dead.

We might even adopt the now-standard concept of death as the irreversible loss of the integrated functioning of the being as a whole. Only now the "being as a whole" whose integration we have in mind is not merely somatic; it is the entire being—mind and body. The permanent collapse of the mind's integration with the body is what might reasonably be thought of as death for all moral, social, and public policy purposes.

We opt for the general formulation that a human is dead when there is irreversible loss of embodied capacity for consciousness. This would make those who have lost all functions of the entire brain dead, of course, but it would also include those who lack consciousness—that is, the permanently comatose, the permanently vegetative, and the anencephalic infant—to the extent that these groups can be identified.

Altered States of Consciousness: A Continuum

We have characterized higher-brain function to refer to consciousness, defined by William James in the 1890s as awareness of self and environment.[15] Consciousness has two clinical components: (1) wakefulness, which is mediated by the ascending reticular activating system of the brain stem, and (2) awareness of self and environment, which is mediated by the cerebral cortex. A coma—an eyes-closed, pathologic state of unresponsiveness—is caused by a structural or metabolic lesion that interferes with the reticular activating system. It is usually transient.[16] A patient in a coma can progress to one of several states: (1) recovery, (2) unresponsiveness, (3) locked-in, or (4) brain death. Patients who remain unresponsive are characterized as in a vegetative state (VS), although the European Task Force on Disorders of Consciousness in 2010 proposed the more neutral term "unresponsive wakefulness syndrome."[17] As the Multi-Society Task Force report on PVS clarified the situation in 1994, those in VS have wakefulness but lack awareness: "Awareness requires wakefulness, wakefulness can be present without awareness."[18] Individuals in VS can be aroused but are not conscious. The VS is considered permanent after three months if it was caused by a hypoxic-ischemic, metabolic, or congenital injury but not until twelve months if it was caused by traumatic brain injury. Some patients who remain unresponsive (or vegetative) will later progress to a minimally conscious state (MCS).

People in MCS have severely altered consciousness but display definite behavioral evidence of conscious awareness.[19] This evidence includes one or more of the following behaviors observed during bedside examination: (1) simple command following, (2) intelligible verbalization, (3) recognizable verbal or gestural yes/no responses (without regard to accuracy), or (4) movements or emotional responses that are triggered by relevant environmental stimuli. The upper boundary of MCS is defined by the recovery of communication or functional use of objects.

To minimize errors in diagnosis and prognosis in patients with altered states of consciousness, standardized neurobehavioral rating scales have been developed. The oldest one is the Glasgow Coma Scale, originally published in 1974.[20] This scale lacks sensitivity to subtle changes of prognostic relevance, which has led to the development of a number of newer instruments that can distinguish between VS and MCS, with the Coma Recovery Scale–Revised (CRS-R) being the measurement of choice.[21]

The problem with the CRS-R and the other scales is that they focus on volitional behavior in patients with severe brain injury who may have fluctuating arousal levels along with impaired sensory and motor functions that can mask signs of consciousness.[22] Some studies suggest a high rate of misdiagnosis (false positives and false negatives) among disorders of consciousness. Luaute and colleagues suggest that erroneous diagnoses of MCS as PVS may reach 40 percent.[23] The natural history and long-term outcomes of MCS have not yet been adequately investigated, although the likelihood of significant functional improvement diminishes over time.[24] Luaute found that more than 70 percent of patients in MCS emerge from minimal consciousness between one and three months after a coma's onset, and some of them recover at least partial independence in activities of daily living. Fewer achieve meaningful recovery if MCS endures from three to six months, although it is not unheard of for an individual to emerge from minimal consciousness after one year or longer.[25] Thus, a time cutoff beyond which the recovery of patients in MCS cannot be expected is impossible to establish.[26] It is common experience that individuals with disorders of consciousness recover their first interaction with the environment through significant emotional stimulation, mostly provided by close relatives or caregivers.[27]

An accurate and reliable evaluation of the level and content of cognitive processing is important for the appropriate management of patients. Objective behavioral assessment of residual cognitive function can be extremely difficult because motor responses may be minimal, inconsistent, and difficult to document. This has led to the use of functional neuroimaging, which has identified some patients with consciousness who fail to show behavioral evidence of consciousness during bedside examination. Two modalities that correspond with active function are [18F]-fluorodeoxyglucose positron emission tomography (FDG-PET) and functional magnetic resonance imaging (fMRI). These modalities work on the basis of glucose consumption by the neurons in the brain. When a person is performing or even thinking about performing a particular task, the regions of the brain that control that task increase their consumption of glucose as a source of energy. That is, glucose metabolism can be seen as a general surrogate marker for conscious experience.[28] PET involves the injection of radioactive elements that localize metabolic activity to particular areas of the brain.[29] An fMRI uses strong magnetic fields to monitor the level of blood oxygenation as a marker of neural activity. It is used more often than PET because of its greater availability and because it poses less risk to subjects.

To the extent that glucose metabolism is a marker for conscious experience, one would expect no metabolic activity in individuals in VS and some activity in individuals with MCS. And yet studies have found some residual activity in some individuals in what we thought was VS.[30] In several rare cases fMRI has demonstrated conscious awareness in patients who are assumed to be vegetative yet who retain cognitive abilities that have evaded detection using standard clinical methods. Similarly, in some patients diagnosed as minimally conscious, functional neuroimaging has revealed residual cognitive capabilities that extend well beyond what is evident even from the most comprehensive behavioral assessment.[31]

Owen and colleagues reported in *Science* in 2006 a case of a woman labeled as being in VS who was able to perform two different mental imagery tasks when instructed.[32] The patient was asked to imagine playing tennis and to imagine walking through a room in her house. The fMRI results were indistinguishable from those for healthy volunteers, leading researchers to conclude that she was imaging those tasks.[33] Others have developed follow-up studies to convert this imagery study into a command-following paradigm in which imagining tennis would be interpreted as yes and walking through the house would be interpreted as no. Monti and colleagues found that five of fifty-four patients (twenty-three in VS and thirty-one in MCS) were able to selectively trigger motor and spatial activation on cue.[34]

The ability to accurately distinguish between MCS and PVS is very important for prognosis and appropriate treatment. It becomes even more critical for those who support higher-brain function definitions of death. Patients in PVS do not interact with their environment, but MCS patients do, such that the former may be eligible for organ donation under a higher-brain definition of death but patients in MCS are not. Given the high number of inaccurate diagnoses, doubt arises.

Measuring the Loss of Higher-Brain Function

If one were to propose a higher-brain function conception of death, the question is, What criteria would be necessary and sufficient for such a declaration, and what tests can determine whether the criteria have been met? Such tests will need to distinguish between individuals with permanent loss of all higher-brain function (those in coma or PVS) and those who may have some consciousness, understood as awareness of the self and the environment.

A higher-brain-function conception of death must address three issues. First, researchers surmise that 30–40 percent of individuals classified as being in PVS are inaccurately labeled. This has important prognostic and diagnostic implications, even more so if one were to adopt a higher-brain-function definition of death. Clearly, those in MCS have some consciousness and would not be dead by a higher-brain definition, whereas those in PVS would be. The high error rate makes one pause.

A second problem is that at the time of the Multi-Society Task Force guidelines on PVS in 1994, most patients in VS had been followed for at most one year. Today, there are more data about late recovery. Estraneo and colleagues followed fifty patients in VS for an average of twenty-six months and found that 20 percent of the sample recovered at least one sign of conscious awareness between fourteen and twenty-eight months after injury, and 24 percent emerged from MCS between nineteen and twenty-five months after injury.[35] Late recovery was more common in younger individuals with a traumatic etiology. This makes it more difficult to identify clear criteria that can be met before one who is in VS is permanently unconscious and can be classified as dead by higher-brain function.

Third, there have been recent developments with medications that have served as a bridge to consciousness. The first case report was published in 2000 in South Africa, where an individual who had been "semicomatose" for three years began to talk and to respond appropriately when treated with zolpidem; he would revert to his semicomatose state when the medication wore off.[36] Since then, there have been other reports involving amantadine and the use of deep thalamic brain stimulation.[37]

Ancillary Tests

First, let us consider whether the ancillary tests for whole-brain death mentioned in chapter 4 can help us identify higher-brain death.

Flat Electroencephalogram

Whereas a flat EEG helps confirm the existence of a permanently nonfunctioning brain, the question remains whether the EEG measures whole-brain function or something more limited. From the scientific evidence, the EEG apparently measures simply the presence of neocortical electrical activity. If this is true, it is quite possible that some brain activity could remain in the presence of a flat EEG. Thus, though EEG activity refutes a claim of irreversible cessation of the functioning of the whole brain, the absence of EEG activity does not necessarily mean the absence of brain function. From the point of view of the higher-brain definition of death, however, could an EEG alone be a measure of death?

The problem with the EEG is that if it measures neocortical activity, it presumably may measure any neocortical activity. Yet we have concluded that the experiential and social integrating function is the essential element in the nature of the human, the loss of which is to be called death. Once again the danger of a false positive diagnosis of living must be raised. The neocortical cells and nerve circuits responsible for the experiential and social integrating function are certainly complex. They would need to include some sensory portions of the cortex, as well as the limbic system and other areas responsible for emotion. Yet is it not theoretically possible that some cortical cells could retain viability and yet the person would be dead in the sense we have discussed? What if, for instance, only motor cortex cells continued to survive through some freak preservation of blood supply to a small area of the cortex or some theoretical artificial perfusion? Whether the EEG would detect activity and whether the existence of only this kind of cortical activity could be distinguished are empirical questions. At the philosophical level, however, for one who sees the human essence to be an embodied experiential and social capacity, the presence of viable motor cells would be of no more significance than the presence of the spinal or cranial reflex arc. Thus, the concept of death being dealt with cannot be reduced without remainder to the criterion of a flat EEG. The irreversible loss of these essential functions may be compatible with the presence of some form of EEG activity. Whether empirical tests can be made to make such a distinction and whether such solely motor cell capacity could ever exist are beyond this discussion.

Blood Flow Studies

The other ancillary tests for the determination of whole-brain death do not do much better than the EEG as a means of measuring higher-brain function. Consider, for example, blood flow studies. Both computed tomography angiography (CTA) and MRA are reliable methods of measuring cerebral blood flow, and the absence of cerebral blood flow is considered an accurate marker of loss of brain function.[38] However, a person may lack upper-brain function and yet still have cerebral blood flow. A false-negative result may occur, for example, if intracranial pressure is relieved by a ventricular drain that restores intracranial blood flow. A CTA may also give false positives in patients with open skull defects who demonstrate minimal cerebral blood flow. An alternative to measuring cerebral blood flow is measuring cerebral perfusion, but these tests may also produce a false negative if there is a cranial defect. These tests may be difficult to interpret.[39]

Neuroimaging

If the older ancillary tests cannot test for higher-brain death, what about the newer modalities of FDG-PET and fMRI scans? Although these modalities are useful for identifying upper-brain function, a negative fMRI does not rule out the possibility that upper-brain function exists. First, many patients in MCS have periods when they are more responsive. Second, some patients may have hearing or other problems that cause them not to receive the sensory input and make the tests unreliable. Third, and most important, a negative test does not fully predict whether the patient will regain these functions in the months to come. The data about moving from VS to MCS suggest that this change can be quite slow, and there is no set time interval after which recovery never occurs. This is particularly true as we learn more about techniques to bridge the arousal and awareness components of consciousness through medication or deep thalamic stimulation.

The problem of doubt returns once again—this time with doubt between the older, broader whole-brain-oriented integrating function and the more limited embodied capacity for consciousness or experiential function. As for us, the case for the concept of the human that sees experiential and social functioning as central is persuasive. The debate about the competing philosophical concepts is complex, much more complex than the original proponents of the older and more naive concept of brain death ever realized. They seemed satisfied to orient attention to brain function, failing to perceive that an irreversible coma and the death of the whole brain were not exactly the same. Moreover, they failed to perceive that neither of these might be exactly the same as the irreversible loss of experiential functions that the Harvard committee's chair indicated were crucial to being alive. Although we personally favor the more limited experiential concept, it is not clear that a test or set of tests can accurately identify those who are irreversibly unconscious and would meet the criteria for higher-brain death. However, if such tests were to be developed, we would support a law that recognizes the debate's complexity and permits the patient or the patient's agent to choose among the plausible death concepts—a position we defend in chapter 6. Our objective in this discussion has been to push beyond the older, simpler whole-brain-oriented concept of death, which is now often used in the literature without careful definition, to achieve a more precise usage of terms. Whether humans die when they lose functions that have a primary locus in the whole brain, in a part of the brain, or in some other organs, it is a human who dies. The choice of the concept of death requires a more precise philosophical choice among these alternatives, and the use of criteria for death, in turn, depends on these philosophical choices.

The Legal Status of Death

Because the literal whole-brain concept of death is coming under increasing criticism, it is important to understand that it remains the legal definition of death in most Western countries. Circulatory criteria for death pronouncement are incorporated into the model law in the United States, so physicians can continue to pronounce death based on loss of circulation. It remains unclear, however, whether loss of circulation is now merely an indirect measure of brain status or is itself intrinsically a sign of loss of life. Moreover, the law states that the loss must be "irreversible," but we have seen that this term is itself ambiguous. Some insist that the loss be physiologically irreversible, but the common practice in routine death pronouncement based on circulatory criteria is that it merely be permanent. Death may be pronounced when no effort will be made to restart circulation, even though in some cases circulation surely could be resumed, at least temporarily, if resuscitative efforts were attempted.

In cases where circulation and other somatic functions are being maintained mechanically, defenders of neurological concepts of death would turn to more direct evidence of the irreversible loss of brain function. As a matter of common practice, the standard criteria for loss of all brain functions continue to be used, even though it is now increasingly clear that certain brain functions (neurohormonal and electrical) can remain when the standard criteria are met.

Unless we insist on revising the criteria for brain-based death pronouncement to measure whether these neurohormonal and electrical activities remain, we are de facto accepting neurological criteria for death that focus on less than literally all brain functions. This raises the question of the legal status of neurological concepts of death that deal with less than the whole brain—the brain-stem and higher-brain concepts.

No jurisdiction in the world has legalized death pronouncement if some brain functions remain. Therefore, higher-brain concepts may be important philosophically but have no legal status. It is striking that at least a large minority of people—philosophers, health professionals, and ordinary laypeople—seem to hold something like a higher-brain concept of death.[40]

Consider the study Laura Siminoff and her colleagues published in 2004.[41] They asked citizens of Ohio to consider three well-described cases: a patient who met the criteria for death of the entire brain, a patient in an irreversible coma (who did not meet brain death criteria), and a patient in PVS. They then asked whether each should be classified as dead. Of the 1,351 who responded, 86 percent considered the first patient dead. (The remainder presumably held something like the circulatory or somatic concept of death.) However, 57 percent also considered the patient in a permanent coma to be dead—a position inconsistent with current law—and 34 percent considered the patient in PVS to be dead. Thus, in the Siminoff study a large majority considered someone dead who had met the standard tests for losing all brain functions, but a majority also considered the comatose (but not brain-dead) patient dead, and a substantial minority considered even the PVS patient—one who was able to breathe on his or her own and went through sleep-wake cycles but was unconscious—to be dead.

Furthermore, we know that an increasing number of scholars and ordinary laypeople would not classify any of these three patients as dead but would nevertheless endorse organ procurement from them in some cases, even though such procurement would end up killing them. That is the view of Miller and Truog.[42] It is also the view of a considerable number of respondents in the Siminoff study—67 percent of those who thought the patient meeting whole-brain-death criteria was alive, 46 percent of those who thought the patient in a permanent coma was alive, and 34 percent of those who thought the patient in PVS was alive. According to this study a majority were willing to procure life-prolonging organs from all three of the patients, although some who were willing to procure (431 of the total of 1,351) favored procuring, believing the patient was dead, and others (305) favored procuring even though they believed the patient was still alive.[43]

The striking conclusion is that among citizens of Ohio in 2004, the majority were willing to procure organs from all three patients.

Only a minority who believed the PVS patient was dead would procure, but another minority who believed the PVS patient was alive would procure and, thus, would be willing to violate the dead donor rule. Although only a minority believed the PVS patient was dead and another minority was willing to procure organs even though they thought the patient was alive, combined these groups make up 55 percent of the respondents.[44]

The confusing public policy problem is that there is no consensus on the definition of death. A large minority, perhaps even a slight majority, favors something like the higher-brain view; another large minority favors the current law, the whole-brain view; and a smaller minority favors the traditional circulatory, or somatic, view. This breakdown seems to have held consistently over many years and among philosophers and theologians, health professionals, and ordinary citizens. The problem, then, is, How can we develop a consistent public policy about what it means to be dead and when life-prolonging organs can be procured? This is the subject of the next chapter.

Notes

1. Goldie WD, Chiappa KH, Young RR, Brooks EB, "Brainstem auditory and short-latency somatosensory evoked responses in brain death," *Neurology* 1981;31(3):248–256; Schrader H, Krogness K, Aakvaag A, Sortland O, Purvis K, "Changes of pituitary homes in brain death," *Acta Neurochirurgica* 1980;52(3–4):239–248. A decade later these facts would resurface in debates about the validity of the definition and determination of brain death. See, for example, Halevy A, Brody B, "Brain death: reconciling definitions, criteria, and tests," *Annals of Internal Medicine* 1993;119(6):519–525. Shewmon also notes similar issues raised by Veatch RM, "The impending collapse of the whole-brain definition of death," *Hastings Center Report* 1993;23(4):18–24; Taylor RM, "Reexamining the definition and criteria of death," *Seminars in Neurology* 1997;17(3):265–270; Truog RD, "Is it time to abandon brain death?" *Hastings Center Report* 1997;27(1):29–37.

2. Halevy and Brody, "Brain death," 520–521.

3. Shewmon DA, "The brain and somatic integration: insights into the standard biological rationale for equating 'brain death' with death," *Journal of Medicine and Philosophy* 2001;26(5):457–478.

4. Latasha Nailah Spears Winkfield (guardian ad litem) v. Frederick S. Rosen, MD, Case No. RG 15760730, Superior Court of the State of California for the County of Alameda, filed November 4, 2015.

5. Bernat JL, "A defense of the whole-brain concept of death," *Hastings Center Report* 1998;28(2):17. See also Bernat JL, "How much of the brain must die on brain death?" *Journal of Clinical Ethics* 1994; 3(1):21–26.

6. See Pallis C, "ABC of brain stem death: reappraising death," *British Medical Journal* 1982;285(6352):1409–1412; Pallis C, "ABC of brain stem death: from brain death to brain stem death," *British Medical Journal* 1982;285(6353):1487–1490.

7. Henry Beecher, the committee's chairman, writing elsewhere: Beecher HK, Dorr HI, "The new definition of death: some opposing views," *Internationale Zeitschrift für klinische Pharmakologie, Therapie, und Toxikologie* [International journal of clinical pharmacology, therapy, and toxicology] 1971;5(2):121.

8. Ibid.

9. Laureys S, Celesia GG, Cohadon F, et al.; European Task Force on Disorders of Consciousness, "Unresponsive wakefulness syndrome—a new name for the vegetative state or apallic syndrome," *BMC Medicine* 2010;8:68. doi: 10.1186/1741-7015-8-68.

10. On personhood, see Lizza JP, *Persons, Humanity, and the Definition of Death* (Baltimore: Johns Hopkins University Press, 2006); on the loss of personal identity, see Green MB, Wikler D, "Brain death and personal identity," *Philosophy and Public Affairs* 1980;9(2):105–133.

11. Green, Wikler, "Brain death."

12. McMahan J, "The metaphysics of brain death," *Bioethics* 1995;9(2): 91–126.

13. Council on Ethical and Judicial Affairs of the American Medical Association, "The use of anencephalic neonates as organ donors," *JAMA* 1995;273(20):1614–1618.

14. Veatch RM, "The death of whole-brain death: The plague of the disaggregators, somaticists, and mentalists," *Journal of Medicine and Philosophy* 2005;30(4):353–378.

15. James W, "The varieties of the religious experience, lecture III: the reality of the unseen," in *New Age, New Thought: William James and the Varieties of Religious Experience*, ed. Miller LL (Denver: Brooks Divinity School, 1999), 51–54.

16. Rubin EB, Bernat JL, "Ethical aspects of disordered states of consciousness," *Neurological Clinics* 2011;29(4):1055.

17. Laureys et al., "Unresponsive wakefulness syndrome."

18. Multi-Society Task Force on PVS, "Medical aspects of the persistent vegetative state," *New England Journal of Medicine* 1994;330(21): 1499–1508.

19. Giacino JT, Ashwal S, Childs N, et al., "The minimally conscious state: definition and diagnostic criteria," *Neurology* 2002;58(3):349–353.

20. Teasdale G, Jennett B, "Assessment of coma and impaired consciousness," *Lancet* 1974;2(7872):81–84.

21. Seel RT, Sherer M, Whyte J, et al.; American Congress of Rehabilitation Medicine, Brain Injury-Interdisciplinary Special Interest Group, Disorders of Consciousness Task Force, "Assessment scales for disorders of consciousness: evidence-based recommendations for clinical practice and research," *Archives of Physical Medicine and Rehabilitation* 2010;91(12):1795–1813.

22. Owen AM, Schiff ND, Laureys S, "A new era of coma and consciousness science," *Progress in Brain Research*, vol. 177, ed. Laureys S, et al. (New York: Elsevier, 2009), 399–411.

23. Luaute J, Maucort-Boulch D, Tell L, et al., "Long-term outcomes of chronic minimally conscious and vegetative states," *Neurology* 2010;75(3):246–252.

24. Giacino et al., "Minimally conscious state," 352.

25. Luaute et al., "Long-term outcomes," 250.

26. Ibid., 247.

27. Formisano R, D'Ippolito M, Risetti M, et al., "Vegetative state, minimally conscious state, akinetic mutism and Parkinsonism as a continuum of recovery from disorders of consciousness: an exploratory and preliminary study," *Functional Neurology* 2011;26(1):15–24.

28. Laureys C, Lemaire C, Maquet P, Phillips C, Franck G, "Cerebral metabolism during vegetative state and after recovery to consciousness," *Journal of Neurology, Neurosurgery and Psychiatry* 1999;67(1): 121–122.

29. Fisher CE, Appelbaum PS, "Diagnosing consciousness: neuroimaging law and the vegetative state," *Journal of Law Medicine and Ethics* 2010;38(2):376.

30. Ibid., 376–377.

31. Owen et al., "New era," 408.

32. Owen AM, Coleman MR, Boly M, Davis MH, Laureys S, Pickard JD, "Detecting awareness in the vegetative state," *Science* 2006;313(5792):1402.

33. Ibid.

34. Monti MM, Vanhaudenhuyse A, Coleman MR, et al., "Willful modulation of brain activity in disorders of consciousness," *New England Journal of Medicine* 2010;362(7):579–589.

35. Estraneo A, Moretta P, Loreto V, Lanzillo B, Santoro L, Trojano L, "Late recovery after traumatic, anoxic or hemorrhagic long-lasting vegetative state," *Neurology* 2010;75(3):246–252.

36. Clauss RP, Güldenpfennig WM, Nel HW, Sathekge MM, Venkannagari RR, "Extraordinary arousal from semi-comatose state on zolpidem: a case report," *South African Medical Journal* 2000;90(1): 68–72.

37. Hirschberg R, Giacino JT, "The vegetative and minimally conscious states: diagnosis, prognosis and treatment," *Neurologic Clinics* 2011;29(4):773–786.

38. Manraj KS, Heran NS, Shemie SD, "A review of ancillary tests in evaluating brain death" *Canadian Journal of Neurological Sciences* 2008;35(4):409–419.

39. Wijdicks EF, "Pitfalls and slip-ups in brain death determination," *Neurological Research* 2013;35(2):169–173.

40. On philosophers, see Haring B, *Medical Ethics* (Notre Dame, IN: Fides, 1973), 131–136; Engelhardt HT, "Defining death: a philosophical problem for medicine and law," *American Review of Respiratory Disease* 1975;112(5):587–590; Veatch RM, "The whole-brain-oriented concept of death: an outmoded philosophical formulation," *Journal of Thanatology* 1975;3(1):13–30; Green, Wikler, "Brain death"; Gervais KG, *Redefining Death* (New Haven, CT: Yale University Press, 1986); McMahan, "Metaphysics of brain death"; Veatch, "Impending collapse"; Whetstine LM, "Bench-to-bedside review: when is dead really dead—on the legitimacy of using neurologic criteria to determine death," *Critical Care* 2007;11(2):308, http://ccforum.com/content/11 /2/208. On health professionals, see Cranford R, Smith D, "Consciousness: the most critical moral (constitutional) standard for human personhood," *American Journal of Law and Medicine* 1987;13(2–3):233–248; Bartlett ET, Youngner ST, "Human death and the destruction of the neocortex," in *Death: Beyond Whole-Brain Criteria*, ed. Zaner RM (Dordrecht: Kluwer Academic Publishers, 1988), 199–215; Machado C, "Is the concept of brain death secure?" in *Ethical Dilemmas in Neurology*, vol. 36, ed. Zeman A, Emanuel LL (London: W. B. Saunders, 2000), 193–212.

41. Siminoff LA, Burant C, Youngner SJ, "Death and organ procurement: public beliefs and attitudes," *Kennedy Institute of Ethics Journal* 2004;14(3):217–234.

42. Miller FG, Truog RD, *Death, Dying, and Organ Transplantation* (New York: Oxford University Press, 2012).

43. Siminoff et al., "Death and organ procurement."

44. Ibid.

The Conscience Clause: How Much Individual Choice Can Our Society Tolerate in Defining Death?

On the morning of March 1, 1994, a blue 1978 Chevrolet Impala pulled next to a van as it began to cross the Brooklyn Bridge. The van was carrying fifteen students from the Lubavitch Hasidic Jewish sect returning from a prayer vigil in Manhattan. As the car neared the van, a lone gunman fired at least five rounds of bullets from two separate semiautomatic weapons into the side of the van while reportedly yelling, "Kill the Jews!" Four students were injured, two critically. One, fifteen-year-old Aaron Halberstam, was "declared brain dead, but he remained on life support."[1]

New York had, at the time, adopted a brain-oriented definition of death through judicial action and administrative regulation of the State Hospital and Planning Council and with the endorsement of the state health commissioner. The regulation read, "Both the individual standard of heart and lung activity and the standard of total and irreversible cessation of brain function should be recognized as the legal definition of death in New York."[2] This would seem to imply that Aaron was dead once the death of his brain was confirmed. However, his parents, following Orthodox Jewish beliefs, insisted that the individual does not die when the brain dies. They would accept only a diagnosis based on respiratory function. The rabbis for the Halberstam family were reported to have said that Aaron should be kept on support systems as long as his heart could beat on its own.[3] The physician, honoring the parents' wishes, refused to pronounce the death. Depending on the interpretation of the state definition and individual hospital policy, this may have been legal. A sentence in the regulation requires each hospital to establish "a procedure for the reasonable accommodation of the individual's religious or moral objection to the determination as expressed by the individual, or by the next of kin or other person closest to the individual."[4]

One can hardly imagine what would have happened if the family had placed its ventilator-dependent, brain-dead, but not-legally-pronounced-dead son in an ambulance and driven him through the Holland Tunnel to New Jersey. When they arrived in New Jersey, they would have been in a jurisdiction with an even more complex legal situation. New Jersey has a whole-brain-oriented definition of death, but the law explicitly permits religious objectors to reject the use of that definition in their own cases, thus making a patient alive until cardiac function ceases irreversibly.[5] If Aaron had been known to object to the whole-brain concept of death, he would clearly have been considered alive in New Jersey, assuming the law applies to minors. The law in New Jersey, however, does not explicitly permit family members to choose a circulatory or somatic definition of death on the basis of their religious beliefs. Thus, unless Aaron's own views were known or the law was extended to permit surrogate decision making, the boy could not have been treated as alive.

The New York case is not the only one that has raised these complex issues surrounding religious and other dissent from the legal definition of death. In California and Florida two additional cases at about the same time pressed the issue. In California on March 27, 1994, two students whose parents lived in Japan were shot in a senseless act of violence and declared "brain dead." According to the report, the students were diagnosed as brain dead, taken off respirators, and then pronounced dead, even though the family was from a culture that at the time did not recognize brain criteria for death pronouncement.[6] The students' parents were not given any discretion to opt for a definition of death that was preferred in their culture.

The sequence of events in this case suggests that the health personnel in California may have been confused. They diagnosed brain death, which alone should have been enough to declare the students dead. However, the hospital personnel did not declare death until after the students had been removed from the respirators (and presumably after their hearts had stopped beating). This delay implies that the personnel pronouncing death did not themselves believe the death of the brain was equivalent to the death of the individual. By contrast, we saw in the Jahi McMath case, described in chapter 3, that by 2013 a patient with confirmed irreversible loss of brain function was pronounced dead in spite of her mother's insistence that she not be considered dead until her heart stopped. In the McMath case the death was pronounced on the basis of brain criteria even though a ventilator continued to support Jahi's heart function.

In Florida in 1994 thirteen-year-old Teresa Hamilton lapsed into a diabetic coma and was subsequently diagnosed as "brain dead." Although Florida, like California, has a law stating that people with dead brains are dead people, Teresa's parents insisted that their daughter was still alive and demanded that she be kept on life support.[7] Although the hospital insisted that the patient was dead and its personnel wanted to stop ventilatory support on the body, the hospital personnel yielded to the family's wishes that Teresa's body be treated as if it were alive. Teresa's parents pressed for a plan to send the girl home on the ventilator without pronouncing her dead. Here the family got its wishes, in spite of the Florida law. Declared brain dead in January 1994, Teresa was moved to her family home in April. Her heart stopped in mid-May, but paramedics revived it. According to Teresa's stepbrother, later that night the family "and her doctor gave up efforts to revive the girl after she again went into heart failure."[8]

The Present State of the Law

Until 1997 the New Jersey law and the New York regulation were unique in the world. In that year Japan adopted an even more complex law that permits brain criteria to be used to pronounce death, but only if the individual while alive has explicitly consented to both the brain-based death pronouncement and organ procurement, and then only if the family also consents.[9] Although many countries have adopted a whole-brain-oriented definition of death, they have done so without any provision for individuals to conscientiously object for religious or other reasons.[10] Similarly, other than Japan, those countries still relying on the more traditional circulatory definition make no provision for their citizens who believe that death should be based on brain function loss. The New York regulation appears to introduce an accommodation based on family objections to a brain-oriented definition, but it actually leaves the details of the policy to individual hospitals. One of the requirements of each hospital's policy must be "a procedure for the reasonable accommodation of the individual's religious or moral objection to the determination as expressed by the individual, or by the next of kin or other person closest to the individual." Thus, if the hospital interpreted reasonable accommodation to include some level of individual physician discretion, one family could express dissent to a physician who is willing to accommodate, while another family may have to deal with a physician who refuses the request to refrain from pronouncing death.[11]

In Singapore in 2013 twenty-two-year-old Swenson Tan was declared dead, and his organs were procured, three weeks after he had lapsed into a coma following an accident in which a van struck the motorcycle he was riding. As his body was wheeled to the operating room for organ removal, his parents and, reportedly, more than thirty friends and family members rallied around him, protesting that they wanted him to be "kept alive."[12] Singapore's Human Organ Transplant Act allows routine organ procurement unless the individual opted out while alive. No provision is made for next-of-kin objection.

The law in most American jurisdictions specifies that if the criteria for measuring the irreversible loss of all brain functions are met, "death shall be pronounced." In other jurisdictions the law reads "death may be pronounced." This seems to imply that the physician could have broader discretion than physicians in New York. The physician could refuse to pronounce based on his or her own personal values, economic considerations, or other factors, in addition to family wishes. Clearly, these laws are defective if they give physicians the legal opportunity to choose whether to pronounce death based on their own values. The problem under consideration in this chapter is whether such discretion could be tolerated by society if the dissent comes from the patient or the patient's next of kin.

The common wisdom has been that such discretion makes no sense. After all, being dead seems to be an objective matter to be determined by good science (or perhaps good metaphysics) rather than by individual conscientious choice. Concern is often expressed that such discretion not only makes no sense but would produce public chaos, leading to situations in which some patients are dead while medically identical patients are alive. Here, we make the case for the legitimacy of a conscientious objection to a uniform definition of death—conscientious objection that permits patients to choose while competent an alternative definition of death, provided that it is within reason and does not pose serious public health or other societal concerns. In cases where patients have not spoken while competent (because, for example, they are infants, children, or adults who simply have not expressed themselves), we argue that the next of kin should have this discretion within certain limits.

Concepts, Criteria, and the Role of Value Pluralism

Understanding our case for conscientious objection requires that we return to a critical point made in earlier chapters: the differences between matters of fact and matters of value in the definition-of-death debate. We argue that matters of value judgment should be open to some level of individual discretion.

The Early Fact-Value Distinction

As we have seen, early in the definition-of-death debate, commentators insisted that a basic distinction be made between two elements of the discussion. What at first appeared to be one question turned out to include at least two separate issues. First, there was a question that seemed primarily scientific: How can we measure that the brain has been irreversibly destroyed (that it has died)? This seems like the kind of question that those skilled in neurology could answer. We have seen in chapter 3 that the neurology community, sometimes aided by others, has offered many sets of criteria, with associated tests and measures, for determining that the brain will never again be able to conduct any of its functions.[13] We have come to understand this as primarily a question for competent medical scientists.[14] (We say "primarily" because we have noted that choosing a set of criteria will involve some decisions that do not rest in science—e.g., decisions about how certain we want to be that brain function loss is irreversible.)

The second question is quite different in character. It asks whether we as a society or as individuals ought to treat an individual with a dead brain as a dead person. The neurology community clearly cannot claim expertise in answering this question. No amount of neurological study could possibly determine whether those with dead brains should be considered dead people. This is a religious, philosophical, ethical, or public policy question, not one for neurological science. When society determines that someone is dead, many social and behavioral changes occur. These are not neurological issues; they are social, normative issues about which all citizens may reasonably voice a position relying on their personal religious, philosophical, and ethical views of the world.

Democratic Pluralism and Value Variation

In a democratic, pluralistic culture, we have great insight into how to deal with religious, philosophical, and ethical controversies about which there are strongly held views and unresolvable controversy. At the level of morality, we agree to tolerate diverse opinions, and we even let a person act on those opinions, at least until their impact on the lives of others becomes intolerable. This is the position we take regarding religious dissent.

Religious and Other Positions

To the extent that the disagreement is a religious or quasi-religious disagreement, toleration of pluralism seems the appropriate course. It permits people with differences to live together in harmony. And at least one major source of division over the definition of death is surely theological. The Halberstam case appears not only to have been caused by anti-Semitic tensions; the moral disagreement about whether to declare Aaron Halberstam dead also has religious roots. Judaism has long been known to include people who oppose brain criteria for death pronouncement—not that all Jews oppose it. Rabbi Moses Tendler, a well-known moral commentator, has supported it.[15] But many Orthodox rabbinical scholars strongly oppose it, maintaining that where there is breath there is life.[16] Some Japanese, influenced by Buddhist and Shinto belief systems, see the presence of life in the whole body, not just in the brain.[17] Native Americans reportedly sometimes hold religious beliefs that oppose a brain-oriented definition of death.[18] Fundamentalist Christians, sometimes associated with the right-to-life movement, and some Catholics focusing on pro-life issues press for a consistent pro-life position by opposing death pronouncement of brain-dead individuals.[19]

Conversely, mainstream Christians, both Protestant and Catholic, support a brain-oriented definition, claiming that being pro-life does not foreclose being clear on when life ends.[20] One Christian theological argument supporting brain-oriented definitions of death starts with the ancient Christian theological anthropology that sees the human as the integration of body and mind or spirit. When the two are irreversibly separated, then the human is gone. This view, as we have seen, places some Christian theologians in the higher-brain camp. These theologians sometimes differentiate themselves from secular defenders of higher-brain concepts. The latter group, under the influence of Derek Parfit, stresses mentalist conceptions of the person that sometimes lead to support for a higher-brain conception that focuses exclusively on the irreversible loss of mental function without concern about the separation of mind from body.[21] By contrast, those working within Christian theology are more likely to insist on the importance of both mind and body.[22]

There are, of course, also some secular people who support a circulatory, or somatic, definition of death. One, now dated, survey found that about two-thirds continued to support such a definition.[23] The only plausible conclusion is that one's definition of death is heavily influenced by one's theological and metaphysical beliefs, along with one's theories of value. We have learned that in a pluralistic society, it is unrealistic to expect unanimity on such questions. Hence, a tolerance of pluralism may be the only way to resolve the public policy debate.

This conclusion seems even more inevitable when one realizes—as we have suggested—that there are not just two or three plausible definitions (whole-brain, circulatory, and higher-brain definitions); there are literally hundreds of possible variants. Some insist on irreversible loss of anatomical brain structure at the cellular level; others, only on irreversible loss of function. Some insist on the loss of cellular-level functions, whereas others insist only on irreversible loss of supercellular functions of integration of bodily function. Some might insist on the loss of all central nervous system functions, including spinal cord function (an early position of Henry Beecher, the chair of the Harvard Ad Hoc Committee),[24] whereas others draw a line between spinal cord and brain. Among higher-brain defenders, there are countless variations on what counts as "higher": everything above the brain stem, the cerebrum, the cerebral cortex, the neocortex, the sensory cortex, and so on. Some, insisting on the loss of all brain functions, ignore electrical functions, limiting their attention to clinical functions.[25] Some are even willing to ignore functions of "nests of cells," claiming that they may be "insignificant."[26] When all the possible variants are combined, there will be a large number of positions; no group is likely to gain the support of more than a small minority of the population. The only way to have a single definition of death is for those with power to coerce others to use their preferred definition. If that single definition were the current "whole-brain" one, with a requirement that literally all functions of the brain must be gone before death is pronounced, the result could be disastrous. No one really believes that every last brain function must be irreversibly lost for a brain to be dead. That would include all electrical functions, all neurohumoral functions, and cellular functions. People's disagreement with this definition would lead to their deviating from it in practice, and this would lead to physician discretion in the absence of a workable official definition of death. Because clinicians would necessarily need to exercise discretion in deciding which functions are to be ignored, patients would be at the mercy of the discretion of the clinician who happens to be present when the question of pronouncing death arises. Even if we were willing to let some ride roughshod over others, it is very unlikely that any one position could gain majority support; in fact, it is unlikely that any single position could come close to a majority. There may be no alternative but to tolerate multiple views.

Constitutional Issues

Once the choice of a definition of death is cast in terms of theological or philosophical issues, the necessity of conscientious choice among the definitions seems more plausible. The constitutional issue of separation of church and state presses us in the direction of accepting definitions with religious groundings. Of course, the constitutional provision prohibiting the establishment of religion does not give absolute freedom of religious action. Many religious beliefs, if acted on, could cause significant harm to others. The "harm to others" principle (or perhaps some more complex social ethical principle, e.g., the principle of justice) necessitates the state's right to limit action based on many belief systems. Snake-handling cults, religious groups that support extremes of corporal punishment for children, religious groups using hallucinogenic drugs, and sects that would practice human and animal sacrifice have all been constrained for the safety and welfare of others.

Nevertheless, the burden on the state to justify interference with religious practice is great. Defenders of the compulsory imposition of a single definition of death on a group of religious conscientious objectors to that definition would need to be supported by evidence of that group's causing significant social harm to other parties. We later argue that such harm cannot be demonstrated. Thus, the New Jersey law authorizes religious objection to the state's default definition of death when there is a religious basis for objecting to the whole-brain definition. Orthodox rabbi Chaim Dovid Zwiebel casts his defense of a conscientious right of Jews to rely on a halachic concept of death (one resembling the circulatory, or somatic, definition) in terms of constitutional rights.[27] He appeals to notions of the free exercise of religion and the right of privacy or personal autonomy.

Problems Limiting Conscientious Objection to Religious Objectors

A state that limits conscientious objection to religious objectors, as New Jersey has done, is likely to face potentially difficult constitutional challenges. New York's regulations, by contrast, carve out a requirement of reasonable accommodation on either religious or moral grounds. We learned from laws permitting religious conscientious objection to service in the military that restricting objection to certain types may be legally indefensible. During the Vietnam War era, some objectors had views that were clearly moral or philosophical, but these objectors had a hard time demonstrating to others that they were religious. Especially if religious is defined as involving belief in a supreme being, many individuals whose objections seemed very similar to religious objections could not qualify. Even members of certain groups often classified as religions could not meet the test of belief in a supreme being; Buddhism, Confucianism, and Native American belief systems all look much like religions, but all fail the supreme being test. Gradually, the restriction of conscientious objection to religious objection was challenged and was found to be discriminatory. The concept of religious objection was gradually broadened to include many belief systems that may not at first appear to be overtly religious.

Some scholars who have studied the New Jersey criterion-of-death law (including some most closely involved with drafting this law) believe that its restriction of the beliefs supporting objection to the brain-oriented definition of death to those that were narrowly religious would be interpreted to also include more broadly moral objections. That at least is the opinion of Robert Olick, an attorney who served as the executive director of the commission that developed the New Jersey law.[28] The only reason that the New Jersey Commission on Legal and Ethical Problems in the Delivery of Health Care and the New Jersey legislature limited its provision to religious objection was political. Even during the debates before passage, some commentators said objections that were not religious, if religion is narrowly construed, would be sustained in a legal challenge.

There are also enormous practical and moral problems with attempts to limit the New Jersey law to religion narrowly construed. At a practical level enforcement officials would need to establish mechanisms for verifying whether an objection was truly religious. A nonpracticing Jew who had a nonreligious objection to a brain-oriented definition of death could cite his religious background, and it would be almost impossible for the state to establish whether his objection was religious. Religious objections have a clear basis for protection in the Constitution, whereas nonreligious objections, despite their logically and morally demanding the same accommodation, do not have the same level of explicit constitutional protection. Nevertheless, morally, the principle of equal respect would seem to require that if religious objections were permitted, then equally sincere and equally deeply held nonreligious philosophical objections would also be equally acceptable. If little is at stake in terms of public interest, little is lost by accepting both on equal terms.

Explicit Patient Choice, Substituted Judgment, and Best Interest

Assuming that the case is made that individuals should be able to exercise religiously or nonreligiously based conscientious choice of an alternative definition of death, should this discretion be extended to surrogate decision makers in the same manner as are terminal illness treatment refusal decisions? The New Jersey law does not explicitly permit parents or other family members to exercise choice on behalf of an incompetent patient. Conversely, the New York regulations do. They follow the pattern established for surrogate decision making in terminal illness. They permit choices "expressed by the individual, or by the next of kin or other person closest to the individual."[29] We see no reason to limit the choice to competent and formerly competent people who have executed advance directives. Surrogates, including those legally designated by power of attorney and those with legal authority as next of kin, have decision-making authority for incompetent patients. We suggest a similar authority for deciding a definition of death. This would require substituted judgment based on what is believed to be the patient's beliefs when they are known and based on best interest judgments when they are not known. In either case an argument can be made that the surrogate should be given a reasonable range of discretion in determining what the patient would have wanted or what is in the patient's best interest.

Consider a formerly competent adult or adolescent who has never formally written a document choosing an alternative definition of death, but who has left an oral record or a lifestyle pattern that appears to the surrogate to favor an alternative definition of death, one differing from the statutory default definition. Aaron Halberstam was returning from an Orthodox Jewish prayer service when he was shot. Assuming he had not written an instruction stating a preference for a circulatory definition of death, should his parents (or other next of kin) have been permitted formally to choose it for him (as, in fact, Aaron's parents did, through the informal decisions in New York)? It appears that he had continued to live the religious life of his parents. There is no reason to doubt that he would choose as they did. Just as the next of kin can presently exercise substituted judgment in forgoing treatment decisions, Aaron's parents likewise should be permitted to choose on his behalf according to the values he is most likely to have held.

Some might claim that this subordinates the interests of the patient or society to the whim of the idiosyncratic beliefs of the next of kin. Below, we argue that there is little at stake for society. As for Aaron's interests, as an unconscious individual he seems to have no explicit contemporaneous interest. If it can be said that he has any residual interests, it surely must be to have his prospective autonomy preserved. Insofar as his parents can deduce what he would have autonomously chosen if he had been able to exercise such judgment, surely they must be permitted, indeed required, to exercise that choice on his behalf.

But suppose we had no idea what Aaron's wishes were about which definition of death should be used in his case. Or suppose he suffered his injury when he was one year old rather than fifteen or twenty-one. Clearly, in this case respecting autonomy is out of the question. The only moral alternative is to use what is considered the best concept of death. But should it be the concept of death considered best by society—perhaps some version of a whole-brain-oriented death, assuming that is the law of the state—or should it be the concept considered best by the patient's next of kin? In the context of forgoing treatment decisions, discretion is now given to the next of kin, under the doctrine of what can be called limited familial autonomy.[30] Just as the individual has an autonomy-based right to choose a definition of death (or a treatment plan), so likewise families are given a range of discretion in deciding what is best for their wards. They select the schooling and religious education that so dramatically shape the system of values and beliefs of the child. They are expected to socialize the child into some value system. In a liberal pluralistic society, we do not insist that familial surrogates choose the best possible value system for their wards; we expect them to exercise discretion, drawing on their own beliefs and values. As long as the ward's interests are not jeopardized too substantially and the interests of the society are not threatened, parents and other familial surrogates should not only be permitted but should actually be expected to make a choice of a definition of death for their wards.

Limits on the Range of Discretion

Clearly, this does not mean that individuals should be able to choose literally any definition of death they please. Someone who has lost all circulatory and brain functions irreversibly, someone whose body can no longer retain cellular integrity, cannot be considered alive, no matter how strongly the individual prefers such a view. There would be serious public health concerns. Likewise, if circulatory functions and brain functions remain so that the individual is conscious, it seems clear that the individual cannot be classified as dead, no matter how strongly the individual holds such a view. (It is an open question whether such an individual should be allowed to choose to forgo life support—or even, if capable, to commit suicide—but no reasonable person would favor a public policy of permitting such a person to be labeled "dead.")

The plausible range of reasonable views includes the three major positions covered in the three previous chapters: the whole-brain, circulatory or somatic, and higher-brain views. We have suggested that the two brain-oriented views both include a substantial minority of the population, at least in Western cultures, but that a persistent minority continues to hold to the circulatory or somatic view. As we have noted, each of these views includes many variants, which means that no one position commands anything like a majority of the population.

Whole-Brain versus Somatic Conceptions of Death

The New Jersey law gives the narrowest of options: between the default whole-brain-oriented definition and the single alternative of a somatic or circulatory definition. That would be a clearly acceptable choice, assuming that there are no significant societal or third-party consequences. The New Jersey plan would seem to offer a minimal range of choice.

The New York regulations are somewhat more open. They require "a procedure for the reasonable accommodation of the individual's religious or moral" views. However, all that is permitted is objection to a determination of death based on the state's preferred definition—that is, the whole-brain view. The clear implication is that the traditional somatic definition is the alternative—that is, the religiously based position of Orthodox Jews, who were the focus of the New York policy discussion. This raises the question of whether conscientious choice can be expanded to include the group of higher-brain concepts of death.

Including Higher-Brain Concepts of Death

We have suggested that more and more people are adopting the position that it is no longer plausible to hold to a literal whole-brain definition of death in which every last function of the entire brain must be dead before death can be pronounced.[31] A case can be made that some higher-brain definitions should be among the choices permitted. Under such an arrangement, a whole-brain definition might be viewed as the centrist view that would serve as the default definition, permitting those with more conservative views to opt for circulatory or somatic definitions and those with more liberal views to opt for certain higher-brain formulations. Of course, this would permit people with brain-stem function, including spontaneous respiration, to be treated as dead. Organs could be procured that otherwise would not be available (assuming the dead donor rule is retained), bodies could be used for research (assuming proper consent has been obtained), and life insurance would pay off.

If higher-brain definitions were among the plausible range of choices and surrogates were permitted to make the choice when there is no clear evidence of the patient's own preference, some might be concerned that this would give surrogates the authority to have their wards treated as dead while some brain and circulatory functions still remain. They see this as posing risks for unacceptable choices, for ending a lingering state of disability, for example. Assuming that the only patients who could be classified as dead by surrogates would be those who have lost all capacity for consciousness—that is, those who have lost all higher-brain functions—the risks to the individual classified as deceased would be minimal. We must keep in mind that surrogates are already presumed to have the authority to terminate all life support for these people, and often, terminating life support means that the patients would soon be dead by most traditional definitions of death. Death would occur within minutes in many cases. The effect on inheritance and insurance would be trivial if patients were simply called dead before medical support was stopped rather than after. Even for those vegetative or comatose patients who had sufficient lower-brain function to breathe on their own, a suspension of all medical treatment would lead to death fairly soon. Adding a higher-brain option to the range of discretion would have only a minimal effect on practical matters and would be a sign that we can show the same respect for the religious and philosophical convictions of those favoring the higher-brain position as we do now in New Jersey and New York for the holders of the circulatory position. If there are actually scores of potential definitions of death within the range from higher-brain to somatic positions, then only a relatively small minority is likely to be in agreement with the default position, whatever it may be. The wise thing to do seems to be to pick some intermediary position and then to permit people to deviate both to somewhat more liberal and somewhat more conservative positions. The choices would probably need to be limited to this range. Both public health and moral problems become severe if the scope of choice is expanded much further.

The Problem of Order: Objections to a Conscience Clause

All of this, of course, depends on the as-yet-undefended claim that there are no significant societal or third-party harms from permitting conscientious objection to a default definition within the range specified. The President's Commission for the Study of Ethical Problems in Medicine and Biomedical and Behavioral Research prepared an important report in 1981 reviewing the definition-of-death debate.[32] In this report the commission examined the circulatory, whole-brain, and higher-brain options. Although the commission's two philosophical consultants on the issue endorsed versions of a higher-brain formulation, the whole commission endorsed the whole-brain position. It gave serious consideration to the higher-brain position before rejecting it for a number of reasons, most of which can be summarized under the heading of problems that would be created for social order.

Death as a Biological Fact

One preliminary objection that was not dwelt on by the President's Commission for the Study of Ethical Problems, but that arises in many discussions of the issue, is the claim that death is not a matter of religious or philosophical or policy choice but rather a matter of biological fact.[33] It is now generally recognized that the choice of a concept of death (as opposed to a formulation of criteria and tests) is really normative or ontological.[34] We are debating as a matter of social policy when we ought to treat someone as dead. No amount of biological research can answer this question at the conceptual level. Of course, many people could still hold that although the definition of death is a normative or ontological question, there is still only one single correct formulation. This seems to be a very plausible position, but we are not discussing the issue of whether there can only be one true definition of death; we are discussing whether society can function for public policy purposes while tolerating differences in beliefs about what the true definition is. Tolerating an Orthodox Jew's or Native American's belief in a definition that is perceived by the rest of society as wrong is no different from having a society tolerate more than one belief about whether abortion or forgoing life support in the living is morally wrong. We are asking whether society can treat people as dead according to their own beliefs rather than whether people are really dead—that is, really conform to some metaphysically correct conception of what it means to be dead—in such circumstances. It is possible to hold that there is one and only one metaphysically correct concept of death but that, out of respect for minority views, society can treat some people who conform to this meaning of death as if they were alive.

The Possibility of Policy Chaos

One of the consistent themes in the criticism of higher-brain definitions, especially with the conscience clause, is that its adoption would lead to policy chaos. Presumably, critics have in mind the stress of health professionals, insurers, family members, and public policy processes, such as succession of the presidency. But a very similar substituted-judgment and best-interest discretion is already granted surrogates regarding decisions to forgo life support on still-living patients. One would think that the potential for abuse and for chaos would be much greater in granting surrogate discretion to decide when to forgo life support. It remains to be seen what chaos would be created from conscientious objection to a default definition of death. If each of the envisioned policy problems can be addressed successfully, then we are left with a religious/philosophical/policy choice for which we should be tolerant of variation if possible and if there are no good social reasons to reject individual discretion. Some of the rebuttal against the charge of policy chaos has already been suggested.

Potential Problems with a Conscience Clause That Includes Higher-Brain Formulations

We need to examine the purported problems that would be created by adopting a conscience clause, especially one that included a higher-brain option. We need to consider problems with the stoppage of treatment, potential abuse of the terminally ill, problems with health and life insurance, the impact on inheritance, spousal issues, the impact on organ transplantation, succession to the presidency, and the effects on health professionals.

Problems with Stoppage of Treatment

One concern is that life-sustaining medical treatment would be stopped on different people with medically identical conditions at different times if conscientious choice among definitions of death is permitted. This assumes, however, that decisions to stop treatment are always linked to pronouncement of death. We now know that normally it is appropriate to consider suspension of treatments in a manner that is decoupled from the question of whether the patient is dead.[35] A large percentage of in-hospital deaths now occur as a result of a decision to stop treatment and let the patient die. Presumably, any valid surrogate who was contemplating opting for a higher-brain definition of death would, if told that this option were not available, immediately contemplate choosing to forgo treatment and let the patient die. In either case the patient would be dead within a short period.

The decoupling of the decision to forgo treatment from that of the pronouncement of death has led some to further decouple what we have called death behaviors, leaving agreed-on points for various behaviors such as initiating grief, procuring organs, and terminating insurance coverage.[36] We should consider such decoupling as it was proposed in the 1970s. There are two reasons to reject it.

First, even if we further decouple death behaviors, different people with different cultural beliefs and values will still consider different times appropriate for each of the behaviors. Some will consider widowhood to begin with the loss of higher-brain function, but others only with the death of the whole brain or the cessation of circulatory and respiratory function. We would still need a conscience clause, but now we would need one for the societally defined point for each of the various death behaviors.

Second, even though some death behaviors surely may plausibly be decoupled from the declaration of death (e.g., deciding to forgo treatment), we should not underestimate the importance of having something resembling a moment of death. Socially and psychologically, we need a moment, no matter how arbitrary, when loved ones can experience a symbolic transition point, at least for a large cluster of these death behaviors. Relatives cannot send flowers one at a time as each moment arrives during a drawn-out process of death involving many different death-related behaviors. Kass won the 1970 argument about whether death was a process or an event.[37] Although dying might be a process, death is not. There must be one defining moment of transition to which at least many of the death-related behaviors may attach.

Abuse of the Terminally Ill

For the same reasons, the risk of abuse of the terminally ill should not be a problem. There could be more concern about a family member dependent on the terminally ill person's pension opting for a somatic definition of death in order to continue receiving a pension or Social Security. Alternatively, one could be concerned that a surrogate would opt for a higher-brain definition in order to reduce hospital expenditures. These, however, seem remote possibilities.

There is also the risk of families (as surrogates) opting for a somatic definition of death when their loved ones have been declared whole-brain dead if the families know that opting for somatic death is possible. They might possibly even lie about the decedent's own wishes. In the emotional intensity of the moment, their denial that the person is dead (with denial as a normal initial psychological response to grief, strengthened by being able to see the body breathing, etc.) may lead them to demand a somatic definition not because either the decedent or even they themselves (if they were to think coolly and rationally about it) actually believe in such a definition, but as a way of (1) practically, keeping their loved one "alive" or (2) psychologically insulating themselves from the reality of the death that has already occurred.

The choice of somatic death may also be an attempt to avoid charges of criminal homicide or manslaughter. Such a case occurred in 1996.[38] Mariah Scoon was a five-month-old infant who had been born prematurely and was declared brain dead in New York in February 1996. Her physician father and lawyer mother, both described as born-again Christians, argued that they did not believe in whole-brain death and wanted to keep Mariah connected to a mechanical ventilator because of their religious faith. Long Island Jewish Medical Center in Queens went to court for the right to shut off the ventilator over the Scoons' objections. Complicating the case was the authorities' suspicion that the cause of death was shaken baby syndrome caused by one of Mariah's parents. Experts were concerned that the longer an autopsy was delayed the less use it would be in assessing the nature and cause of Mariah's brain injuries. The court battle was rendered moot when John Cardinal O'Connor, the Roman Catholic archbishop of New York, helped arrange for Mariah's transfer to St. Vincent's in New Jersey. Mariah's heart stopped in March 1996. An autopsy was quickly done and provided the evidence necessary to find Dr. Scoon guilty of manslaughter two years later.

These abuses are all possible, but the same risks currently exist when family members or other surrogates make decisions to forgo life support. Families presently could continue life support in order to keep receiving a pension or could forgo it in order to avoid costs. They could continue it because of their psychological need to keep their loved one alive or their desire to avoid a homicide charge. Falsifying the patient's wishes would be a violation of respect, but keeping a patient alive for psychological reasons already happens from time to time. Professional caregivers have means of confronting these issues and usually can bring about a satisfactory resolution. Moreover, there is no record of a person's attempting to manipulate whether a patient is classified as living in New Jersey, where the option of a somatic definition is available. If the problem did arise, the procedures currently available for review of suspected patient abuse would be available so that the surrogates could be removed from their role, just as they would be now if they refused life support for a patient for their own financial gain.

The cases of Jahi McMath and Aden Hailu make clear that even if the law requires a single brain-based definition of death, a determined family can insist that the support of bodily functions continue.

Health Insurance

There exists a potential impact on health insurance if someone chooses a definition of death that would have the effect of making someone live longer—if, for instance, a somatic definition were chosen. (If some version of a higher-brain definition were chosen, the effect would more likely be a savings in health insurance.) There is good reason to believe that the effect on health insurance would be minimal. A relatively small number of people would actively make a protreatment choice because of their preference for a somatic definition or any alternative that would require longer treatment. The small costs would probably be justified in the name of preserving respect for individual freedom on religious or philosophical matters. If the problem became significant, a health insurance policy could address the problem. Any health insurance policy must have some limits on coverage. Cosmetic surgery is usually not covered, and there are often limits on the number of days of inpatient care for psychiatric services. Many marginal procedures, including longer days of stay in the hospital, are rejected. If insurers were worried about unfair impact on the subscriber pool if their funds were used to provide care for patients without brain function who had selected a somatic definition of death, they could simply exclude coverage for care for living patients with dead brains or offer such coverage as an additional option at an increased premium. The patient and caregivers would be left in the position in which they presently find themselves when they want a treatment not funded by insurance coverage. They could self-pay, buy supplemental insurance, rely on charity, or accept the reality that not all desired medical interventions are available to all people.

Life Insurance

The concern of life insurance companies is exactly the opposite. Insisting on a somatic definition would simply delay payment, which would be in the insurer's interest; however, selecting a higher-brain definition would make the individual dead sooner, potentially quite a bit sooner. However, most living people with dead brains die fairly soon, either because such patients are hard to maintain or because an advance directive or surrogate opts for termination of treatment. In the case of patients who prefer a higher-brain definition of death, if they are not permitted to choose it, in all likelihood they will have advance directives forgoing life support or family surrogates will refuse that support, so these patients will die at more or less the same time that they would have if they had been permitted to choose a higher-brain definition.

Inheritance

As in the case of pensions and life insurance, some surrogate might be inclined to manipulate the timing of death to gain an inheritance more quickly. This could lead to choosing a higher-brain definition. However, as we have seen, the same surrogate already has the power to decline medical treatment, which would theoretically expose the patient to similar risks, and such cases are exceedingly rare. If a surrogate is suspected of abusing a patient by choosing an inappropriate concept of death, such a surrogate can always be challenged and removed. If one compares the risk of abuse from surrogate discretion in deciding to forgo treatment with that from deciding on a variant definition of death, surely the discretion in forgoing treatment is more controversial and more subject to abuse. Yet this has not proved to be a significant problem.

Marital Status

Another social practice that can be affected directly by the timing of a death is the marital status of the spouse. Spouses may want to retain their status as spouses rather than become widows or widowers for various psychological and financial reasons. Or they may want to become widows or widowers so that they can get on with their lives. Conceivably, some may be ready to remarry. For example, a spouse who had been caring for a patient in PVS for years may have already separated psychologically from his or her mate even though the patient was not actually dead. This person could be ready to remarry, which could be done legally once the spouse was deceased. This problem seems quite far-fetched, but it could happen. Such spouses would probably already have contemplated refusing life support and could be removed as inappropriate surrogates if it is clear that they are motivated for non-patient-centered reasons that lead to inappropriate decisions.

Organ Transplants

One significant impact of the definition of death is the availability of organs for transplant. A person who insists on a somatic or circulatory definition of death would not be able to donate organs when heart function remains, even though brain function has ceased. However, anyone who selected a somatic definition of death would be unlikely to be an organ donor if he or she were forced to be pronounced dead on the basis of brain criteria in any case. Conversely, a person who chose to be considered dead even though lower brain function remains would be a potential organ source. Those who wanted to have organs procured when their higher-brain functions were irreversibly lost potentially could have their organs procured earlier by selecting a higher-brain definition. As long as this was limited to cases where an active choice was made in favor of the higher-brain formulation, it is hard to see why there would be strong objections. Alternatively, with the evolution of donation after circulatory death protocols (which we discussed in chapter 4), individuals who prefer the higher-brain definition could become organ donors by refusing life support to the point of death, followed by organ procurement. The outcomes would be similar, except that in the latter scenario, the donor would be forced to participate in the use of a concept of death that he or she rejected and the quality of the organs might be jeopardized.

Many people have pressed for a law authorizing organ procurement from living anencephalic infants.[39] The AMA Council on

Ethical and Judicial Affairs (CEJA) temporarily endorsed such a view in 1995.[40] But it seems that CEJA must have been muddled. If we mean by "death" nothing more than being in a condition when it is appropriate for others to engage in death-associated behaviors and we include procuring organs in the list of such behaviors, then anyone who is an appropriate candidate for procuring so-called life-prolonging organs is dead.[41] By this logic, if the AMA council really believed it was acceptable to procure organs from an anencephalic infant with remaining brain-stem function, then, to be consistent, it should have claimed that such anencephalic infants are already dead (or, more accurately, have never been alive). In effect CEJA adopted a version of a higher-brain-oriented definition of death, and if it wanted to be consistent, it should really have claimed that it is acceptable to procure organs from anencephalic infants because they are dead (or have never been living, in the social policy sense of the term). In fact, CEJA quickly reversed its endorsement of anencephalic infant organ procurement, making its position once again consistent with a whole-brain view of the definition of death.[42]

Succession to the Presidency

Another potential implication of choosing an alternative definition of death is that succession to the presidency or to other roles could be affected. In the United States the vice president is automatically elevated to the presidency upon the death of the president. Similar policies affect monarchies, where the successor is automatically made king. A president who chose a circulatory definition of death could thereby end his or her term of office at a different time than one who chose a whole-brain or higher-brain definition. Because, in certain circumstances, one can retain cardiac function for years, the succession of the vice president could be delayed for a long time.

Obviously, this reflects a flaw in the succession law. Under present law a permanently vegetative president is not dead and there would be no automatic succession. But as soon as PVS is diagnosed, there should be immediate succession regardless of whether the president is dead. One could imagine a person who is next of kin being pressured to choose a definition with an eye toward timing the succession. That could happen now in an effort to delay the succession of the governorship in New Jersey. It could happen elsewhere if discretion were permitted. But the possibility of this happening seems extremely remote. The Twenty-Fifth Amendment to the Constitution provides a mechanism for the temporary assumption of the presidency, but once a president is known to be permanently incapacitated, he or she clearly should be replaced.

The Effect on Health Professionals

A final potential problem with authorizing conscientious choice is the possible effect on the health professionals who are providing care for the patient. Nurses will be required to suffer potential emotional stress at having to continue care or cease care at a time they believe inappropriate. Physicians will face similar problems. But this is hardly a problem unique to a choice of a definition of death. Some living patients or their surrogates refuse life-supporting therapy before the nurse or physician believes it is appropriate. Yet these health professionals are simply obliged to stop according to the laws of informed consent and the right to refuse treatment. More recently, professionals have been disturbed about requests for care that the clinicians deem "futile." Patients who insisted on not being pronounced dead until their heart stopped could conceivably insist on hospital-based treatment even though their brains were dead. That is potentially the situation in New Jersey now and was temporarily the situation in California during the McMath case. But the responsibility of the health professional to deliver care deemed futile against his or her will is already a matter of considerable controversy.[43] It will need to be resolved whether or not other states adopt the New Jersey conscience clause. Texas has adopted a law permitting physicians to unilaterally stop life support on still-living terminally ill patients when certain conditions are met.[44] Most patients demanding such care are clearly not dead by any definition. The resolution could be the same for patients with dead brains as it is for terminally ill or vegetative patients, or it could be different. The law could determine, for instance, that conscious patients would have a right of access to normatively futile care (perhaps with the proviso that they have independent funding) but that permanently unconscious patients or those with dead brains would have no right of access. In any case the impact on caregivers is not a problem unique to patients who might exercise an option for an alternative definition of death. If the concern is about the cost of additional treatment rather than the psychological effects of having to care for the patient, this is more of an insurance issue. As we have argued previously, the additional cost is likely to be a minor burden on the health care system, and if it turned out to be a problem, laws could be passed requiring those who choose a somatic definition to buy supplemental insurance or a policy could be developed that makes clear that living patients with dead brains are not entitled to long-term ventilator support or other intensive care unit therapies at public expense.

Implementation of a Conscience Clause

The procedural implementation of a conscience clause would require some additional planning, but the problems would not be novel. Most of the potential problems are addressed in the existing Patient Self-Determination Act and required request laws. The Patient Self-Determination Act requires the hospital staff to inquire about the existence of an advance directive upon a patient's admission to a hospital and provide assistance in executing an advance directive if the patient desires. The required request laws require that the next of kin be notified of the opportunity to donate organs in suitable cases. The most plausible way to record a choice of something other than a default concept of death would be in one's advance directive. That is the kind of document that ought to be on the minds of those caring for a patient who is near death. An addition specifying a choice of an alternative concept of death would be easy; it would be crucial in the case of those who are writing an advance directive demanding that life support continue even though the brain is dead. It would be a simple clarification in the case of one asking that support be forgone when the patient is permanently unconscious. A sentence choosing a higher-brain concept of death (and perhaps donating organs at that point) would be a modest addition.

Whether the new definition-of-death laws authorizing a conscience clause should also impose a duty on health professionals to notify patients or their surrogates of alternative concepts of death is a pragmatic question that would need to be addressed. Just as Orthodox Jews presently carry the burden of notifying others of their requirements for a kosher diet and Jehovah's Witnesses carry the burden of notifying others about refusal of blood transfusions, so those with alternative concepts of death would plausibly carry that burden. Something akin to the subjective standard for informed consent would apply. According to this standard, health professionals, when they negotiate a consent, are required to inform the patient of what the patient would reasonably want to know, but they are not expected to surmise all the patient's unusual views and interests. According to this approach, health professionals would be expected to initiate discussions on alternative definitions of death only when they knew or had reason to know that the patient plausibly would be interested in such a discussion. A clinician who knew that his or her patient was an Orthodox Jew and knew that many Orthodox Jews prefer a more traditional concept of death would have such an obligation, but would not if he or she had no reason to believe that the patient might be inclined toward an alternative concept.

Some might claim that adding a conscience clause is unnecessary because only a small group of people would favor an alternative. In fact, a not insignificant number seem to prefer a more traditional circulatory or respiratory concept of death (Orthodox Jews, Native Americans, Japanese, and others who are still committed to the importance of the heart or lungs). If a higher-brain-oriented concept of death were among the options, a much larger minority would have an interest in exercising the conscience clause. In fact, there have been a number of court cases and anecdotal reports of families objecting to the use of whole-brain-based concepts. It seems reasonable to assume that these represent only a fraction of the total number of cases in which patients or families would prefer either a more traditional or a more innovative concept of death.

Even if it could be shown that few people would care enough about the concept and criteria of death used to pronounce them or their loved ones dead, this is still an important issue to clarify. It is important if the rights of only a small minority are violated. It is also important as a matter of conceptual clarity and of principle. The knee-jerk revulsion to a conscience clause for alternative concepts of death probably reflects a lingering belief that deciding when someone is dead is a matter of biological fact (for which individual conscience seems irrelevant). But insisting that the choice of a concept of death be treated as a matter of philosophical and theological dispute seems to follow naturally once one realizes the true nature of the issues involved. Getting people to think about why a conscience clause is appropriate for this issue has an important teaching function and serves to respect the rights of minorities on deeply held religious and philosophical convictions.

Conclusion

Once one grasps that the choice of a definition of death at the conceptual level is a religious/philosophical/policy choice rather than a question of medical science, the case for granting discretion within limits in a liberal pluralistic society is a very powerful one. There seems to be no basis for imposing a unilateral normative judgment on the entire population when the members of the society are clearly divided. When one realizes that there are many variants and that no definition is likely to receive the support of a majority, pluralism appears the only answer. Having a state choose a default definition and then granting individuals a limited range of discretion within the limits of reason seems to be the only defensible option. There is no reason to limit this discretion to religiously based reasons and no reason why familial surrogates should not be empowered to use substituted judgment or best-interest standards for making such choices, just as they presently do for forgoing treatment decisions that determine even more dramatically the timing of death. A default with an authorization for conscientious objection seems the humane, respectful, fair, and pragmatic solution.

Notes

1. "Man charged in shooting of Jewish students," *New York Times*, March 3, 1994.

2. "Failure of brain is legal 'death,' New York says," *New York Times*, June 19, 1987.

3. "In hospital hallways, family and friends pray for victims," *New York Times*, March 3, 1994.

4. New York Codes, Rules and Regulations, "Determination of death," title 10, section 400.16, http://w3.health.state.ny.us/dbspace /NYCRR10.nsf/56cf2e25d626f9f785256538006c3ed7/8525652c 00680c3e8525652c00634c24?OpenDocument&Highlight=0,400.16.

5. New Jersey Declaration of Death Act, signed April 8, 1991; it reads, in part: "The death of an individual shall not be declared upon the basis of neurological criteria . . . of this act when the licensed physician authorized to declare death, has reason to believe, on the basis of information in the individual's available medical records, or information provided by a member of the individual's family or any other person knowledgeable about the individual's personal religious beliefs that such a declaration would violate the personal religious beliefs of the individual. In these cases, death shall be declared, and the time of death fixed, solely upon the basis of cardio-respiratory criteria."

6. "Slaying suspects share a past marred by crime," *New York Times*, April 1, 1994.

7. "Florida hospital seeks to end life support of comatose girl," *New York Times*, February 13, 1994; "Brain-dead Florida girl will be sent home on life support," *New York Times*, February 19, 1994.

8. Associated Press, "Brain-dead teen dies of heart failure," *AP News Archive*, May 13, 1994, www.apnewsarchive.com/1994/Brain-Dead -Teen-Dies-of-Heart-Failure/id-00b533297e549575b1b1770e4daf1ddf.

9. Law Concerning Human Organ Transplants (Law No. 104 in 1997).

10. In a 2002 survey Wijdicks found legal standards for organ transplantation in fifty-five of eighty countries for which he located information. To make matters more complicated, in some countries for which there was no legal standard, there existed nevertheless practice guidelines for determining brain death (implying that they may be used without further legal authorization). A total of seventy of eighty countries have such guidelines. Thus, a number of countries for which information was available (e.g., Barbados, Ecuador, Guatemala, Honduras, Egypt, Ghana, Syria, Armenia, China, Pakistan, and Vietnam) had neither law nor guidelines. In at least some of these countries, reports exist of death pronouncement based on brain criteria in spite of the absence of law or practice guidelines. See Sui WG, Yan Q, Xie SP, et al., "Successful organ donation from brain-dead donors in a Chinese organ transplantation center," *American Journal of Transplantation* 2011;11(10):2247–2249. Because Wijdicks was able to find no information one way or the other for more than 100 countries, it is clear that the international situation regarding brain death is quite complex and confusing. (See Wijdicks EFM, "Brain death worldwide: accepted fact but no global consensus on diagnostic criteria," *Neurology* 2002;58:20–25.)

In 2015 Wahlster and colleagues distributed an electronic survey globally to physicians with expertise in neurocritical care, neurology, or related disciplines. Responses were received from 94 of 123 countries. Of 91 complete responses, 63 (70 percent) reported a legal provision and 70 (77 percent) reported an institutional protocol for brain death. There was wide variability in requisite examination findings, with over half of respondents deviating from the AAN criteria. There were legal barriers in the practice of brain death determination in some of the most populous countries (e.g., India, China, and Egypt). (See Wahlster S, Wijdicks EF, Patel PV, et al., "Brain death declaration: practices and perceptions worldwide," *Neurology* 2015;84[18]:1870–1879.) This study did not ask what was done if a family rejected brain death criteria. However, in 2014 members of critical care professional societies worldwide participated in a consensus development process using a Delphi process. (See Sprung CL, Truog RD, Curtis JR, et al., "Seeking worldwide professional consensus on the principles of end-of-life care for the critically ill: the Consensus for Worldwide End-of-Life Practice for Patients in Intensive Care Units [WELPICUS] study," *American Journal of Respiratory and Critical Care Medicine* 2014;190[8]:855–866.) Responses came from thirty-two countries. Consensus was prospectively defined as greater than 80 percent agreement. If a statement received less than 80 percent agreement, a revised statement could be considered. With respect to brain death, 84 percent of participating countries' respondents agreed that "families that do not accept brain death should receive an explanation that their loved one has been declared dead medically and that under these circumstances all life-sustaining treatments are discontinued" (p. 860). Similarly, a revised statement achieved 83 percent support; it read: "If the surrogate decision maker or family does not accept brain death and objects to the discontinuation of the ventilator or other therapies sustaining organ function, the physician and institution should discontinue all therapies sustaining organ function. Therapies may be continued for a limited time to help families accept the death of their relative" (p. 860). A smaller majority were willing to accommodate family wishes; 68 percent of respondents agreed with a revised statement: "If the surrogate decision maker or family who do not accept brain death have their wishes respected to continue therapies sustaining organ function because, under these circumstances, the Law requires health care professionals to continue therapies sustaining organ function, the 'patient' does not have to remain in an ICU if allowed by hospital policy" (p. 860).

11. New York Codes, Rules and Regulations, "Determination of death."

12. "Man declared brain dead after being hit by van at Hougang," *Singapore Seen*, March 11, 2013, http://singaporeseen.stomp.com.sg/this -urban-jungle/man-declared-brain-dead-after-being-hit-by-van-at -hougang.

13. Harvard Medical School, "A definition of irreversible coma: report of the Ad Hoc Committee of the Harvard Medical School to Examine the Definition of Brain Death," *JAMA* 1968;205(6):337–340; Task Force on Death and Dying, Institute of Society, Ethics, and the Life Sciences, "Refinements in criteria for the determination of death: an appraisal," *JAMA* 1972;221(1):48–53; "Report of the medical consultants on the diagnosis of death to the President's Commission for the Study of Ethical Problems in Medicine and Biomedical and Behavioral Research," in *Defining Death: Medical, Legal and Ethical Issues in the Definition of Death*, ed. President's Commission for the Study of Ethical Problems in Medicine and Biomedical and Behavioral Research (Washington, DC: US Government Printing Office, 1981), 159–166; Cranford RE, "Minnesota Medical Association criteria: brain death—concept and criteria, part I," *Minnesota Medicine* 1978;61(9):561–563; Law Reform Commission of Canada, *Criteria for the Determination of Death* (Ottawa: Ministry of Supply and Services, 1981); "An appraisal of the

criteria of cerebral death: a summary statement. A collaborative study," *JAMA* 1977;237(10):982–986.

14. More recent analysis has challenged the blatant fact-value dichotomy implied in this separation of the criteria question as one for medical science and the concept question as one of religious, philosophical, or public policy. See Veatch RM, *Death, Dying, and the Biological Revolution*, rev. ed. (New Haven, CT: Yale University Press, 1989), 43–44.

15. Tendler MD, "Cessation of brain function: ethical implications in terminal care and organ transplant," in *Brain Death: Interrelated Medical and Social Issues*, ed. Korein J (New York: New York Academy of Sciences, 1978), 394–397; Veith FJ, Fein JM, Tendler MS, Veatch RM, Kleiman MA, Kalkinis G, "Brain death, I: a status report of medical and ethical considerations," *JAMA* 1977;238(15):1651–1655.

16. Bleich JD, "Establishing criteria of death," *Tradition* 1972;13(3):90–113; Bleich JD, "Neurological criteria of death and time of death statutes," in *Jewish Bioethics* (New York: Sanhedrin Press, 1979), 303–316; Rosner F, "The definition of death in Jewish law," *Tradition* 1969;10(4):33–39.

17. Kimura R, "Japan's dilemma with the definition of death," *Kennedy Institute of Ethics Journal* 1991;1(2):123–131.

18. President's Commission, *Defining Death*, 41.

19. Byrne PA, O'Reilly S, Quay PM, "Brain death: an opposing viewpoint," *JAMA* 1979;242(18):1985–1990.

20. For Protestants, see Hauerwas S, "Religious concepts of brain death and associated problems," *Brain Death: Interrelated Medical and Social Issues*, vol. 315 of *Annals of the New York Academy of Sciences*, ed. Korein J (New York: New York Academy of Sciences, November 1978), 329–338; Potter RB, "The paradoxical preservation of a principle," *Villanova Law Review* 1968;13:784–792; Ramsey P, "On updating death," in *Updating Life and Death*, ed. Cutler DR (Boston: Beacon Press, 1969), 31–53. For Catholics, see Haring B, *Medical Ethics* (Notre Dame, IN: Fides, 1973), 131–136.

21. Parfit D, *Reasons and Persons* (Oxford: Clarendon Press, 1984); Green MB, Wikler D, "Brain death and personal identity," *Philosophy and Public Affairs* 1980;9(2):105–133.

22. Ramsey P, *The Patient as Person* (New Haven, CT: Yale University Press, 1970), xiii; Veatch, *Death, Dying*, 42.

23. Charron WC, "Death: a philosophical perspective on the legal definitions," *Washington University Law Quarterly* 1975;1975(4):979–1008.

24. Harvard Committee, "Ad hoc report," talks of spinal reflexes. Raymond Adams, a Harvard neurologist involved in the ad hoc committee explains that he chose "complete unresponsivity and areceptivity [which] would include everything, even spinal reflexes . . . [to avoid] an error that permitted the inclusion of any reversible cases." Laureno R, *Raymond Adams: A Life of Mind and Muscle* (New York: Oxford University Press, 2009), 95. By 1970 Beecher no longer advocated for the inclusion of spinal reflexes. See Beecher HK, "Definitions of 'life' and 'death' for medical science and practice," *Annals of the New York Academy of Sciences* 1970;169(2):471–474.

Although Beecher and US guidelines no longer require the absence of spinal reflexes for the determination of death, a global survey of brain death practices and perceptions published in 2015 found that "a relatively large proportion (23%) of respondents stated that they would require absent spinal reflexes to determine brain death" (Wahlster et al., "Brain death declaration," 1877).

25. Ashwal S, Schneider S, "Failure of electroencephalography to diagnose brain death in comatose patients," *Annals of Neurology* 1979; 6(6):512–517.

26. Bernat JL, "How much of the brain must die on brain death?" *Journal of Clinical Ethics* 1992;3(1):21–26.

27. Zwiebel CD, "Accommodating religious objections to brain death: legal considerations," *Journal of Halacha and Contemporary Society* 17(1):59–68.

28. Robert Olick, personal communication, October 23, 1996; Olick RS, "Brain death, religious freedom and public policy," *Kennedy Institute of Ethics Journal* 1991;1(4):275–288. Also see Goldberg CK, "Choosing life after death: respecting religious beliefs and moral convictions in near death decisions," *Syracuse Law Review* 1984;39(4):427–468.

29. New York Codes, Rules and Regulations, "Determination of death."

30. Veatch RM, "Limits of guardian treatment refusal: a reasonableness standard," *American Journal of Law and Medicine* 1984;9(4):427–468.

31. Veatch RM, "The whole-brain-oriented concept of death: an outmoded philosophical formulation," *Journal of Thanatology* 1975;3(1):13–30; Engelhardt HT, "Defining death: a philosophical problem for medicine and law," *American Review of Respiratory Disease* 1975;112(5): 587–590; Bernat, "How much of the brain must die"; Haring, *Medical Ethics*, 131–136.

32. President's Commission, *Defining Death*.

33. For a discussion, see Gervais KG, *Redefining Death* (New Haven, CT: Yale University Press, 1986), 45–74; Lamb D, "Diagnosing death," *Philosophy and Public Affairs* 1978;7(2):144–153; Becker LC, "Human being: the boundaries of the concept," *Philosophy and Public Affairs* 1975;4(2):334–359.

34. For normative, see Veatch, *Death, Dying*; for ontological, see Green, Wikler, "Brain death."

35. The general problem of decoupling of behavioral correlates of pronouncing death is the subject of Fost N, "The unimportance of death," in *The Definition of Death: Contemporary Controversies*, ed. Youngner SJ, Arnold RM, Schapiro R (Baltimore: Johns Hopkins University Press, 1999), 161–178.

36. Brody B, "How much of the brain must be dead?" in *Definition of Death*, 71–82; Fost, "Unimportance."

37. The debate was published in *Science*. See, Morison RS, "Death: process or event?" *Science* 1971;173(3998):694–698; Kass LR, "Death as an event: a commentary on Robert Morison," *Science* 1971;173(3998): 698–702.

38. This paragraph is based on several reports about the case of Mariah Scoon published in the newspapers. See Bruni F, "Medical certainty, legal limbo," *New York Times*, February 28, 1996; Bruni F, "Hospital ordered to keep brain-dead baby alive," *New York Times*, February 29, 1996; Bruni F, "Brain-dead baby's heart stops despite ventilator," *New York Times*, March 14, 1996; Donohue P, "Dad guilty of shaking baby Mariah to death," *New York Daily News*, April 4, 1998; Sengupta S, "Doctor guilty in '96 death of daughter," *New York Times*, April 4, 1998.

39. Harrison MR, Meilaender G, "The anencephalic newborn as organ donor," *Hastings Center Report* 1986;16(2):21–23; Fletcher J, Robertson J, Harrison M, "Primates and anencephalics as sources for pediatric organ transplants," *Fetal Therapy* 1986;1(2–3):150–164; Walters JW, Ashwal S, "Organ prolongation in anencephalic infants: ethical and medical issues," *Hastings Center Report* 1988;18(5):19–27.

40. American Medical Association, Council on Ethical and Judicial Affairs, "The use of anencephalic neonates as organ donors," *JAMA* 1995;273(20):1614–1618.

41. Of course, some organs (single kidneys and liver lobes) can be procured from living people. We do not insist on people being declared dead in these cases. It is considered appropriate behavior even for the living, assuming that proper consents have been obtained.

42. American Medical Association, Council on Ethical and Judicial Affairs, "The use of anencephalic neonates as organ donors—reconsidered. Unpublished meeting proceedings," AMA Interim Meeting, December 1995, Chicago, IL. This was incorporated into AMA opinion 2.162—anencephalic neonates as organ donors, *AMA Code of Medical Ethics*, March 1992, www.ama-assn.org/ama/pub /physician-resources/medical-ethics/code-medical-ethics/opinion2162 .page.

43. Bosslet GT, Pope TM, Rubenfeld GD, et al.; American Thoracic Society Ad Hoc Committee on Futile and Potentially Inappropriate Treatment, American Thoracic Society, American Association for Critical Care Nurses, American College of Chest Physicians, European Society for Intensive Care Medicine, Society of Critical Care, "An official ATS/AACN/ACCP/ESICM/SCCM policy statement: responding to requests for potentially inappropriate treatments in intensive care units," *American Journal of Respiratory and Critical Care Medicine* 2015;191(11):1318–1330; Truog RD, "Counterpoint: The Texas advance directives act is ethically flawed: medical futility disputes must be resolved by a fair process," *Chest* 2009;136(4):968–971; Fine RL, "Point: The Texas advance directives act effectively and ethically resolves disputes about medical futility," *Chest* 2009;136(4):963–967; McCabe MS, Storm C, "When doctors and patients disagree about medical futility," *Journal of Oncology Practice* 2008;4(4):207–209.

44. Texas Health and Safety Code, chap. 166, subchapter A, §166.052. Of note, at the time we are writing, there is a court case in which the family of David Christopher Dunn is challenging the decision by Houston Methodist Hospital that Dunn's care is futile. The court already granted a temporary restraining order barring the hospital from ending life-sustaining care. (See Schencker L, "Family fights Texas law allowing providers to end life-sustaining care," *Modern Health Care*, November 29, 2015, www.modernhealthcare.com/article/20151129 /NEWS/151129929.)

7

Crafting a New Definition-of-Death Law

Changing current law to conform to the suggestions made in the preceding chapters is a complex endeavor and should be done with deliberate speed—but it should be done. Three changes to the current definition of death are needed: (1) the higher-brain-function notion should be incorporated, (2) some form of the conscience clause should be incorporated, and (3) the concept of irreversibility should be clarified.

Incorporating the Higher-Brain-Function Notion

Present law makes people dead when they have lost all functions of the entire brain. It is uniformly agreed that the law should incorporate only this basic concept of death, not the precise criteria or tests needed to determine that the whole brain is dead. That is left up to the consensus of neurological experts and is likely to change as technology advances.

All that would be needed to shift to a higher-brain formulation is a change in the wording of the law to replace "all functions of the entire brain" with some relevant, more limited alternative. There are at least three options: references to higher-brain functions, cerebral functions, or consciousness. Although we could simply change the wording to state that an individual is dead when there is irreversible cessation of all higher-brain functions, that poses a serious problem. We are now suffering from the problems created by the vagueness of the phrase "all functions of the entire brain." Even though referring to "all higher-brain functions" is conceptually correct, it would be even more ambiguous. The revision would lack the needed specificity.

The new phrase could be given substance by referring to the irreversible loss of cerebral functions, but we have already suggested two problems with this wording. Just as we now know there are some isolated functions of the whole brain that should be discounted, so there are probably some isolated cerebral functions that most would not want to count either. For example, if, hypothetically, an isolated nest of cerebral motor neurons were perfused so that if stimulated the body could twitch, that would be a cerebral function, but not a significant one for determining life any more than a brain-stem reflex is. Second, in theory some really significant functions, such as consciousness, might someday be maintainable even without a cerebrum—if, for example, a computer could function as an artificial center for consciousness. The term "cerebral function" adds specificity but is not satisfactory.

The language that seems best if integration of mind and body is what is critical is the "irreversible cessation of the capacity for consciousness." This is, after all, what the defenders of the higher-brain formulations really have in mind. (If someone were to claim that some other "higher" function is critical, that alternative could simply be plugged in.) In chapter 5 we actually endorsed a concept of death related not only to consciousness but also to the capacity for social interaction. We went on, however, to suggest that we could envision no cases in which the presence of consciousness would not also permit social interactions. Likewise, we cannot envision one who possesses the capacity for social interaction without consciousness. The two, we argued, were coterminous. We are therefore content to propose a higher-brain definition of death based on the irreversible loss of the capacity for consciousness. We noted previously that medical experts need to make some evaluative judgments about what appear to be matters of scientific fact. With this qualification acknowledged, we will leave the specifics of the criteria and tests for measuring the irreversible loss of the capacity for consciousness up to the consensus of neurological expertise.[1] If the community of neurological expertise claims that the irreversible loss of consciousness cannot be measured, so be it. We will have at least clarified the concept and set the stage for the day when it can be measured with sufficient accuracy.

The Conscience Clause

A second significant change in the definition of death would be the incorporation of the conscience clause. This clause would permit individuals, when competent, to execute documents choosing alternative definitions of death that are, within reason, not threatening to the significant interests of others. Although New Jersey law permits choosing only a heart-oriented definition as an alternative to a whole-brain position, and the Japanese law permits limited options for choosing a whole-brain definition as an alternative to a circulatory definition, our proposal is to choose a default definition, perhaps a whole-brain default, and permit individuals to choose a reasonable alternative, say, a somatic or higher-brain view. Assuming some version of a whole-brain formulation—adjusted to acknowledge that minor, cellular electrical activity and probably also hormonal regulatory functions should be ignored—as a default definition would permit choosing either somatic or higher-brain-oriented (consciousness-based) definitions as alternatives.

As we have indicated, New Jersey law presently permits only competent adults to execute such conscience clauses. This, of course, excludes the possibility of parents choosing alternative definitions for their children. We argue that just as legal surrogates have the right to make medical treatment decisions for their wards, provided the decisions are within reason, so too should they be permitted to choose alternative definitions of death, provided the individual had never expressed a preference. Although New Jersey law tolerates only explicitly religiously based variation, we would favor variation based on any conscientiously formulated position.

As a shortcut the law could state that patients who had opted for the consciousness-based definition who had clearly irreversibly lost consciousness because their heart and lung function had ceased could continue to be pronounced dead according to criteria measuring heart and lung function. It would have to be made clearer than in the present Uniform Determination of Death Act that measuring circulatory function is simply an alternative means for measuring the loss of consciousness. We see no reason to continue including the alternative forms of measurement in the legal definition itself. We would simply leave those to the criteria articulated by the consensus of experts. As long as heart and lung function had stopped long enough to make a return of consciousness impossible, the individual could be pronounced dead based on higher-brain function loss.

Similarly, for those who rely on the default (modified whole-brain) definition, as long as heart and lung function had stopped long enough to make impossible the return of any brain function (adjusted to exclude trivial electrical and hormonal functions), the individual could be pronounced dead based on whole-brain function loss.

Clarification of the Concept of Irreversibility

One final change needs to be made regardless of whether the higher-brain concept and the conscience clause are added to the law defining death. In chapter 2 we summarized the controversy over the notion of irreversibility included in the law. It has sometimes been understood to mean that the critical function—brain function, circulatory function, or higher-brain function, depending on the concept one chooses—physiologically could not be restarted. Because this implies that the physiological substrate for the function has been destroyed, this version of irreversibility is sometimes called "physiological irreversibility."

Alternatively, irreversibility has been understood to mean "will never be restarted." Sometimes the critical function could be restarted but will not be, perhaps because needed technology or those with the requisite skills are not present or perhaps because someone has made a valid decision that resuscitation will not be attempted. For example, a patient suffering a terminal illness may have on record an advance directive refusing further resuscitation. In such a case it would be illegal and immoral to attempt resuscitation. After one has waited long enough to rule out the restarting of function spontaneously (autoresuscitation), one could conclude that the stoppage is irreversible, in the sense that no one will try to reverse the function loss. This is sometimes called "legal irreversibility" or merely "permanent" function loss.

The original model definitions of death were typically not clear on which meaning of irreversible was intended. One might be inclined to opt for the more conservative notion of physiological irreversibility. Doing so, however, conflicts with the traditional practice of medicine. Consider an elderly patient with metastatic cancer who has an advance directive refusing life support who then suffers a cardiac arrest. Typically, a physician present, after having established the absence of a circulatory function, will simply pronounce death. No resuscitation will be attempted, and there will be no waiting period for the body's tissues to decline to the point that circulation could not be restored. There is simply no point in waiting. In other words, traditionally, we have measured irreversibility using the "will not be restored" definition rather than the "physiologically cannot be restored" version.

Now that the issue is clear, a model law needs to specify which meaning is intended. We recommend the traditional notion of "will not be restored"—that is, the function morally or legally cannot be restored. This is standard practice today, and it should be made explicit in the model law. We do so in the text we recommend.

A Proposed New Definition of Death
for Public Policy Purposes

This leads to a proposal for a new definition of death, which would read as follows:

There shall be three acceptable definitions of death: (1) irreversible loss of all functions of the entire brain, excluding cellular-level and hormonal regulatory functions; (2) irreversible loss of consciousness; and (3) irreversible loss of circulatory function. A determination of any of these for the purpose of pronouncing death shall be made in accordance with accepted medical standards. Definition (1) shall be the default definition according to which an individual shall be declared dead unless he or she, while competent, or a designated surrogate, legal guardian, or next of kin, as specified below, has asked that the individual be declared dead according to definition (2) or (3). "Irreversible" shall be taken to mean that a valid decision has been made not to attempt reversal, and there is an empirical basis for believing there will be no spontaneous reversal. An individual who has chosen one of these alternatives shall be declared dead according to the definition that he or she has chosen. However, no individual shall be treated as dead for public policy purposes unless he or she has sustained irreversible cessation of all consciousness and no individual shall be treated as alive for public policy purposes if he or she has irreversibly lost all circulatory and respiratory functions.

Unless an individual has, when competent, selected a definition of death to be used for his or her own death pronouncement, a designated surrogate, legal guardian, or next of kin (in that order) may do so relying on substituted judgment, insofar as information is available about the patient's own wishes. If no such information is available, the decision maker shall rely on a best-interest determination. The definition selected by the individual, designated surrogate, legal guardian, or next of kin shall serve as the definition of death for all legal purposes. If no such alternative is selected, then the default definition shall be used.

Some have proposed that an additional paragraph prohibiting a physician with a conflict of interest (e.g., an interest in the organs of the deceased) from pronouncing death. We are not convinced that paragraph is needed, however.

Conclusion

It has been puzzling why what at first seemed like a rather minor debate over when a human was dead should have persisted as long as it has. Many thought the definition-of-death debate was a technical argument that would be resolved in favor of the more fashionable, scientific, and progressive brain-oriented definition as soon as the old romantics attached to the heart died off. It is now clear that something much more complex and more fundamental is at stake. We have been fighting over the question of who has moral standing as a full member of the human moral community, a matter that forces on us some of the most basic questions of human existence: the relation of mind and body, the rights of religious and philosophical minorities, and the meaning of life itself.

We are left with two options if we do not adopt the definition we propose including a conscience clause. First, we could revert to a circulatory or somatic definition of death, following the arguments of Shewmon, Miller and Truog, and the minority of the US President's Council on Bioethics.[2] We would then need to face the question of whether certain prohibitions encapsulated in the dead donor rule should be abandoned. For example, we could choose to permit organ procurement in certain limited cases before death, as endorsed by Miller and Truog, who have argued for the legitimacy of organ procurement in cases of individuals who have decided to withdraw from life support and who have also acted to donate their organs. That would, in effect, mean abandoning the dead donor rule and permitting intentional, active killing of this group of patients—killing by organ procurement. We think those drastic social policy changes are unlikely, although a 2015 survey suggests that a majority of the US public may support such a policy change.[3] The alternative, if we are to revert to a circulatory or somatic definition of death, is to hold to the dead donor rule and permit the procurement of life-prolonging organs only by donation after circulatory death—this would mean a substantial loss of organs, but it is a plausible position if one is committed to the circulatory definition of death. If that option is chosen, major social and public policy changes would be required, including amending all state and national definition-of-death laws to repeal the brain-based positions. That would be a major social undertaking.

The second alternative is to opt for some version of a higher-brain definition. Individuals would be declared dead when they irreversibly lose the capacity for consciousness. A large minority of the population in Western culture appears to hold this position, but only a minority. Adopting it without a conscience clause would impose a still-controversial definition on a large number of people. We are not certain whether some version of the higher-brain-oriented definition of death will be adopted in any legal jurisdiction anytime soon, but we are convinced that the now old-fashioned whole-brain-oriented definition of death is becoming less and less plausible as we realize that no one really believes that literally all brain functions must be irreversibly lost in order for an individual to be dead. Unless some public consensus is expressed in state or federal law conveying agreement on exactly which brain functions are insignificant, we are all vulnerable to a slippery slope in which private practitioners choose for themselves exactly where the line should be drawn from the top of the cerebrum to the caudal end of the spinal cord. There is no principled reason to draw it exactly between the base of the brain and the top of the spine. Better that we have a principled reason for drawing it. To us, the principle is that for human life to be present—that is, for the human to be treated as a member in full standing of the human moral community—there must be integrated functioning of mind and body. This means some version of a higher-brain-oriented formulation relying on the presence of a capacity for consciousness and social interaction. At the same time, we understand that not everyone shares this view. We see no significant, unavoidable social costs in permitting people to choose, based on their beliefs and values, from among the plausible definitions—the somatic, whole-brain, and higher-brain views.

Notes

1. Even determining the criteria for measuring irreversible loss of capacity for a brain function such as consciousness involves fundamentally nonscientific value judgments. The community of neurologists, for example, would need to choose a probability level at which the prediction of irreversibility can be made. They would have to add nuanced meaning to the terms critical for the enterprise. They would have to assume certain concepts in their work. Neurologists are not experts in any of these matters. In theory the lay community could disagree with the consensus of neurological experts, and in disputes over these matters, the lay population would have a legitimate claim to have their preferences and assumptions used in choosing the criteria for measuring irreversible loss of consciousness. For example, if the lay population wanted greater levels of statistical significance than the community of neurological experts, there is no rational reason why the neurologists' choice of a significance level should prevail. See Veatch RM, *Death, Dying, and the Biological Revolution*, rev. ed. (New Haven, CT: Yale University Press, 1989), 41–44; Veatch RM, "Consensus of expertise: the role of consensus of experts in formulating public policy and estimating facts," *Journal of Medicine and Philosophy* 1991;16(4):427–445.

2. Shewmon DA, "The brain and somatic integration: insights into the standard biological rationale for equating 'brain death' with death," *Journal of Medicine and Philosophy* 2001;26(5):457–478; Miller FG, Truog RD, *Death, Dying, and Organ Transplantation* (New York: Oxford University Press, 2012); US President's Council on Bioethics, *Controversies in the Determination of Death: A White Paper by the President's*

Council on Bioethics (Washington, DC: US President's Council on Bioethics, 2008).

3. Nair-Collins M, Green SR, Sutin AR, "Abandoning the dead donor rule? a national survey of public views on death and organ donation," *Journal of Medical Ethics* 2015;41(4):297–302.

INDEX

Academy of Medical Royal Colleges, 48–49
advance directives, 24, 74–75, 122, 133, 137–38, 151
American Academy of Neurology (AAN), 5, 48, 49, 51, 56–59, 141n10
American Academy of Pediatrics, 47–50
American Bar Association (ABA), 4–5, 44
American Medical Association (AMA), 4–5, 19, 44, 134–35

Beecher, Henry, 43, 50, 51, 58, 89–91, 144n24
Bernat, James, 5–6, 89, 90
Boucek, Mark M., 79–82
brain: and anoxic damage, 47, 53, 57, 66–67, 72; and blood flow tests, 46–49, 102; and body, 95–96; and cellular activity, 53, 56, 101–2, 118, 119, 149, 152; and criteria for function loss, 42–53, 55–58, 59, 69, 88, 104, 117; destruction of, 45–53; and determination of death, 4–7, 13–16, 58, 68, 104, 147; electri-

cal activity in, 45, 50, 52–53, 88, 101, 104, 118, 119, 149, 150; essential functions of, 6–7, 20–21, 90–96, 154–55; and higher-brain, 3–4, 21, 30, 60–61, 99–100, 150; and hormones, 4, 50, 55–56, 59, 88, 104, 149, 150, 152; and integrative functions, 21–23, 32, 43–44, 50–51, 59, 68, 69, 76, 82–85, 89, 91, 94, 96, 118; and irreversible function loss, 2–3, 15, 16, 21–22, 32, 39, 43–53, 67, 69–71, 73, 76–78, 88, 101–4, 118, 124; and reflexes, 20, 49, 50–51, 59, 61, 144n24; and whole-brain function loss, 3–4, 5, 20–21, 42–53, 88–90, 116, 125, 147, 152
brain-stem death, 59–61, 89, 104

Capron, Alex, 68, 69
cardiac arrest: and Aden Hailu, 59; and brain's blood flow, 69; and circulation, 70–71, 76; and clinical death, 23; and heart starting again, 1, 23, 25, 35n16; and irreversibility, 1, 23, 24–25,